THE *Skinny*

SLOW COOKER

Student

RECIPE BOOK

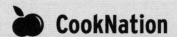 CookNation

THE SKINNY SLOW COOKER STUDENT RECIPE BOOK

DELICIOUS, SIMPLE, LOW CALORIE, LOW BUDGET, SLOW COOKER MEALS FOR HUNGRY STUDENTS. ALL UNDER 300, 400 & 500 CALORIES

ISBN 978-1-909855-74-8

A CIP catalogue record of this book is available from the

British Library

DISCLAIMER

This book is designed to provide information on the dishes that can be cooked in an electric slow cooker appliance. Results and or timings may differ dependant on the product used.

Some recipes may contain nuts or traces of nuts. Those suffering from any allergies associated with nuts should avoid any recipes containing nuts or nut based oils.

This information is provided and sold with the knowledge that the publisher and author do not offer any legal or other professional advice.

In the case of a need for any such expertise consult with the appropriate professional.

This book does not contain all information available on the subject, and other sources of recipes are available.

This book has not been created to be specific to any individual's requirements.

Every effort has been made to make this book as accurate as possible. However, there may be typographical and or content errors.

Therefore, this book should serve only as a general guide and not as the ultimate source of subject information.

This book contains information that might be dated and is intended only to educate and entertain.

The author and publisher shall have no liability or responsibility to any person or entity regarding any loss or damage incurred, or alleged to have incurred, directly or indirectly, by the information contained in this book.

All recipes are calorie counted below 500 calories. We do not reccomend these recipes to anyone under 18 years old, is eldery, pregnant or breastfeeding. If in doubt consult your doctor or health professional.

CONTENTS

MEAT DISHES 47

VEGGIE DISHES 67

INTRODUCTION

The Skinny Slow Cooker Student Recipe Book should be an essential part of any student checklist.

If you are reading this book the chances are you've either been gifted a slow cooker by a relative and are looking for some inspiration to make uni and college meal times tastier, easier, cheaper and healthier. Or perhaps you've turned a corner and, fed up with boring dinners every night, you're looking to inject some life into your meals. You might even be on a diet or managing your weight. Whatever the reason The Skinny Slow Cooker Student Recipe Book should be an essential part of any student checklist.

Inspiration for this book came when we noticed our original Skinny Slow Cooker Recipe Book - Delicious Recipes Under 300, 400 and 500 Calories was a top 10 best selling cookbook according to TheNationalStudent.com. We've taken all that's best about that book – great tasting meals that are simple, no fuss and low calorie and tailored it to be the perfect kitchen companion for any student. It's packed with tasty, low budget, low calorie dinners and snacks. All you need to do is set and go.

We know that students by and large are far more health conscious than they used to be and that the staple diet of beans on toast, kebabs or packet pasta just aren't on the menu any more. Let's face it, you've opted to educate yourself above and beyond high school, capable of understanding relatively complex theories and can write an essay or two – following our slow cooker recipes – even with no previous kitchen experience - is a breeze. Preparation time is kept to a minimum, ingredients are simple to source, cheap and lots of the store cupboard ingredients can be use over and over again. Using a slow cooker is the best way of cooking when you are a student. Once you've prepped your ingredients they all go in the slow cooker and you just set the controls and leave it to work its magic. Get on with your studying, hook up with your mates and when you return you'll be met with a kitchen filled with amazing aromas and a healthy, balanced, low calorie dinner cooked to perfection.

Our skinny slow cooker recipes all serve 4. There are a few reasons for this.

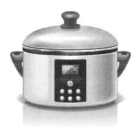

- Most slow cookers are sized to cook for more than 1-2 people.
- Cooking for 4 means you have 3 more meals left over which you can freeze and reheat for another day. Perfect!
- Cooking for friends is even better. Invite your mates round and share!

KITCHEN STUFF

Lets face it...most student kitchens aren't particularly well equipped – an oven, microwave if you're lucky and a few burnt pots and pans. Still it's a kitchen and luckily for you, using a slow cooker with our recipes, there are only a few additional pieces of kitchen equipment that will make prep time easier.

- Non-stick saucepan
- Non-stick frying pan
- Set of sharp knives – one for cutting veg, one for dicing meat, one for smaller jobs like garlic or chilli.
- Can opener, peeler, grater, garlic crusher
- Wooden spoons, ladle and potato masher
- Mixing bowl
- Hand whisk
- Colander – great for washing salads, draining rice
- Chopping boards – ideally 2 – one for meat and one for veg
- Measuring jug
- Tablespoon, dessert spoon, teaspoon
- Potato peeler

Asking family to buy some of these items is a great idea. Most mums will be more than happy to help set you up to help you eat properly. For some items you can go to one of the many bargain-style high street shops like Poundland, Home Bargains and B&M to pick up things like measuring jugs and wooden spoons for next to nothing.

HYGIENE

We're not talking personal hygiene, as important as that is, but food hygiene. It's really important if you want to avoid getting sick. It's not just about paying attention to 'use by' dates on packaging but things like keeping raw and cooked food separate and allowing food to cool properly before refrigerating or freezing. Read on to learn the basics of food hygiene in the kitchen and avoid being featured in the next series of Ramsay's Kitchen Nightmares:

- Wash your hands before preparing any food.
- Wash your fruit & veg before using. This will remove any possible remnants of pesticides that may or may not have been used in their production. Plus think about how many other people have picked up and examined your piece of veg in the supermarket before you bought it! Use cold running water to rinse.
- Raw meat should be covered, refrigerated and placed on the lowest shelf in

the fridge to prevent any juices dripping onto other food.
- Keep food covered – especially in warmer weather when bugs are in abundance.
- Wash your work surfaces – ideally before, as well as after preparing food. Use hot soapy water.
- Wash tea towels and dish cloths regularly. They can be a perfect breeding ground for germs.
- Allow food to cool properly and as quickly as possible (ideally within 90 minutes) then put in the fridge and use within a couple of days or freeze).
- Defrost meat in the fridge ideally overnight. Don't leave it sitting out in direct sunlight all day – you're asking for a stomach-ache.

SKINNY FRIDGE ESSENTIALS

To keep calories low, all our recipes apply the skinny factor – that is replacing high calorie/high fat ingredients with lower calorie, healthier alternatives. So if watching your calories is on the agenda when it comes to meal times, then you should always use and have the following in your fridge:

* Low fat Greek yogurt
* Semi skimmed/ half fat milk
* Reduced fat cheese
* Low fat/unsaturated 'butter' spreads (like olivio or flora)
* Low cal cooking oil spray
* Low fat cream/ crème fraiche

STORE CUPBOARD ESSENTIALS

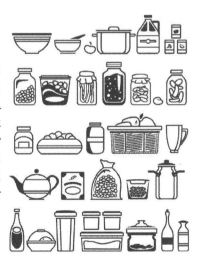

The following is a list of really handy ingredients to have in your cupboard that you will use over and over again when cooking. Most have a very long shelf life and don't need to be kept in the fridge. It's by no means essential to get them all. We know cooking as a student needs to be as low budget as possible so don't rush out and blow your weekly budget in one go. Try picking up a few items now and again and shop in budget stores like Lidl and Aldi. Better still when you're next home at mum or dad's, raid the cupboard and take home a stash of everything you can get your hands on. See our 'How To Shop' guide on page 11.

- Tomato puree (you can usually substitute with ketchup as a last resort)
- Tomato passata
- Mixed tinned/canned beans (chickpeas, cannellini etc – you can mix and match on most recipes)
- Lemon juice
- Plain flour
- Cornflour
- Chicken & vegetable stock
- Garlic (lots of recipes call for fresh garlic but 'lazy' garlic or garlic powder will work too)
- Fresh ginger (some recipes call for fresh ginger but 'lazy' ginger or ginger powder will work too)
- Honey

- Dried spices : Papirka, Turmeric, cumin, Ginger, Coriander, chilli powder, chilli flakes, garam masala Chinese five spice powder
- Curry powder
- Dijon mustard
- Dried Italian herbs : sage, thyme, basil, rosemary, oregano (remember a lot of these herbs are interchangeable, you don't need them all)
- Soy Sauce
- Worcestershire sauce
- Tinned chopped tomatoes
- Brown sugar
- Salt & pepper

COOKING TECHNIQUES

If you've ever watched any celebrity chef on TV or glanced at a cookbook then you will no doubt have come across a never-ending list of techniques to apply to create the perfect dish – basting, folding, beating, marinating, kneading, simmering, resting….the list goes on. The really great thing about using a slow cooker is that very few of these techniques are needed. Yes there is a certain amount of prep: like frying some onions or browning some mince but after that the slow cooker does everything for you. It's really that simple, which means fewer kitchen utensils used and less washing up!

Here's an explanation of the most common techniques we refer to in our skinny recipes:

Sauté: This just means gently frying in a little oil to release the flavours and soften.

Reduce: This is when you simmer liquid until part of it evaporates and you have less liquid. This creates a more intense flavour.

Marinate: This is when ingredients are covered in sauce/marinate prior to cooking to flavour the flesh.

Flouring Meat: Meat is sometimes covered with flour as a sauce/stew thickener. The easiest way to do this is to put the meat and flour in a bag and shake.

Browning/Sealing Meat: Cooking the surface of the meat at a high temperature gives the meat a deeper flavour. Brown in batches if needed as you don't want too many pieces in the pan at the same time.

Grate: Use a hand grater to move the vegetable (peel first), cheese or fruit up and down the jagged surface of the grater. Some graters have different sides for different textures.

Deseeding Chillies & Peppers: Slice lengthways, remove the by scraping with a knife or spoon and remove the white membranes inside.

Deseeding Butternut Squash: Use a peeler to get rid of the skin. Cut off the top and bottom. Slice in half lengthways and use a spoon to scoop out the seeds and stringy bits.

Season: This just means adding some salt and pepper to add flavour and balance the taste.

Combine: This means using a spoon to gently bring the ingredients together without breaking anything apart with hard stirring.

Crushed: Use a garlic press to crush the peeled garlic clove. Finely chop if you don't have one.

Peeling: All vegetables/fruit should be peeled unless stated otherwise. Vegetables with 'ends' like carrots and courgettes should have these sliced off.

HOW TO SHOP

This might sound like a strange concept, but when you are cooking on a budget there are a few basic rules that should try to stick to in order get the best value out of your shopping.

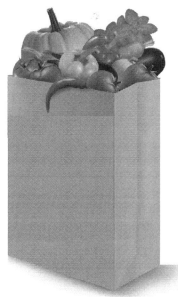

- Don't shop when you're hungry! Buying food when you're famished will result in over priced, probably unhealthy choices.
- Don't shop when you are short of time. Again you will most likely make bad choices unless you know exactly what you are looking for.
- Take your time cruising the aisles. There may be alternatives to choose from which are better value. Remember that most supermarkets will usually place the most expensive items at eye level. Look up and down the shelves.
- Choose supermarket 'own' brands but be careful that any 'everyday' or value' items aren't high in salt and sugar.
- Buy food that can be frozen.
- Buy food that is frozen. Frozen veg, meat, fish are all good.
- Buy tinned fruit and veg. These still count towards your five-a-day but last longer. Just watch out for tinned fruit that is in 'syrup' – look for 'juice' instead.

- Buy fruit and veg that is in season. These tend to be cheaper when not imported.
- Don't go overboard on fresh items. Only buy what you will use or can freeze. Perishable items like fruit and veg only keep for a few days.
- Shop at the end of the day when many items may be reduced to clear BUT check the use by dates first.
- Look out for '2 for 1' promotions on items like pasta and rice that last for a long time. Where possible go for wholegrain pasta and brown rice.
- Go for cheaper cuts of meat. The slow cooker is at its best when it tenderises tougher and usually cheaper cuts of meat.

PREPARATION

All the recipes should take no longer than 10-15 minutes to prepare. Browning the meat will make a difference to the taste of your recipe, but if you really don't have the time, don't worry - it will still taste great.

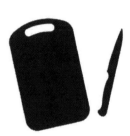

All meat and vegetables should be cut into even sized pieces unless stated in the recipes. Some ingredients can take longer to cook than others, particularly root vegetables, but that has been allowed for in the cooking time. Meat should be trimmed of visible fat and the skin removed.

SLOW COOKER TIPS

- All cooking times are a guide. Make sure you get to know your own slow cooker so that you can adjust timings accordingly.
- Read the manufacturers operating instructions as appliances can vary. For example, some recommend preheating the slow cooker for 20 minutes before use whilst others advocate switching on only when you are ready to start cooking.
- Slow cookers do not 'brown' meat. While this is not always necessary, if you do prefer to brown your meat you must first do this in a pan with a little low calorie cooking spray.
- Don't be tempted to regularly lift the lid of your appliance while cooking. The seal that is made with the lid on is all part of the slow cooking process. Each time you do lift the lid you will need to increase the cooking time.
- Removing the lid at the end of the cooking time can be useful to thicken up a sauce by adding additional cooking time and continuing to cook without the lid on. On the other hand if perhaps a sauce it too thick removing the lid and adding a little more liquid can help.
- Always add hot liquids to your slow cooker, not cold.
- Do not overfill your slow cooker.
- Allow the inner dish of your slow cooker to completely cool before cleaning. Any stubborn marks can usually be removed after a period of soaking in hot soapy water.
- Be confident with your cooking. Feel free to use substitutes to suit your own taste and don't let a missing herb

or spice stop you making a meal - you'll almost always be able to find something to replace it.

· A spray of one calorie cooking oil in the cooker - before adding ingredients - will help with cleaning or you can buy liners.

ABOUT COOKNATION

You might also like some of our other recipe books in the skinny range including a number of slow cooker cookbooks. Go to the end of the book to browse all our titles, head over to **Amazon** or visit **www.cooknationbooks. com**

CookNation is the leading publisher of innovative and practical recipe books for the modern, health-conscious cook.

CookNation titles bring together delicious, easy and practical recipes with their unique approach - making cooking for diets and healthy eating fast, simple and fun.

With a range of #1 best-selling titles - from the innovative 'Skinny' calorie-counted series, to the 5:2 Diet Recipes Collection - CookNation recipe books prove that 'Diet' can still mean 'Delicious'!

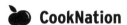 **CookNation**

Skinny
SLOW COOKER
Student
CHICKEN DISHES

CHICKEN & OLIVE STEW

330 calories per serving

Ingredients

- 4 chicken breasts, each weighing 175g/6oz
- 1 tbsp plain flour
- 1 onion, peeled & sliced
- 2 garlic cloves, crushed
- 1 red or orange pepper, deseeded & sliced
- 1 tsp dried mixed herbs
- 2 tbsp pitted olives, sliced
- 250ml/1 cup hot chicken stock
- 1 tin chopped tomatoes (400g/14oz)
- 2 handfuls tenderstem broccoli (200g/7oz), roughly chopped
- Low cal cooking oil spray
- Salt & pepper to taste

Method

1 Turn the slow cooker on so that it starts heating up.

2 Cut the chicken breasts in half and season well.

3 Place the chicken in a plastic bag with the flour and give it a good shake until well coated.

4 Meanwhile place a non-stick frying pan on a low heat and gently sauté the onions, garlic & peppers in a little low cal spray for a few minutes until softened.

5 Tip the onions and peppers out of the pan onto a plate.

6 Add some more oil to the pan, increase the heat and quickly brown the chicken pieces for a minute or two to seal the meat.

7 Put everything, except the broccoli, in the slow cooker. Combine well, cover with the lid and leave to cook on low for 5-6 hours or high for 3-4 hours.

8 Add the broccoli about 45 minutes before the end of cooking time. Make sure the chicken is cooked through. Season and serve.

CHEFS NOTE

This is great served with a light green salad or crusty bread.

SWEET GARLIC CHICKEN & PEPPERS

315 calories per serving

Ingredients

- 1 onion, sliced
- 4 garlic cloves, crushed
- 3 red peppers, deseeded & sliced
- 4 chicken breasts, each weighing 175g/6oz
- 2 tsp cornflour, dissolved into a little warm water to make a paste
- 1 tbsp honey
- 500ml/2 cups hot chicken stock
- Low cal cooking oil spray
- Salt & pepper to taste

Method

1 Turn the slow cooker on so that it starts heating up.

2 Place a non-stick frying pan on a low heat and gently sauté the onions, garlic & peppers in a little low cal spray for a few minutes until softened.

3 Tip the onions and peppers out of the pan onto a plate.

4 Add some more oil to the pan, increase the heat and quickly brown the chicken breasts for a minute or two to seal the meat.

5 Put everything in the slow cooker and gently combine. Cover with the lid and leave to cook on low for 5-6 hours or high for 3-4 hours.

6 Make sure the chicken is cooked through. Season and serve.

CHEFS NOTE
Bulk up this dinner by adding some straight-to-wok noodles to the slow cooker 10 minutes before serving if you like.

PINEAPPLE SALSA CHICKEN

360 calories per serving

Ingredients

- 1 small tin pineapple chunks (200g/7oz), reserve the juice
- ½ red chilli, deseeded & finely chopped
- 1 tbsp freshly chopped coriander
- 1 tbsp soy sauce
- 4 chicken breasts, each weighing 175g/6oz
- 1 tbsp plain flour

- 1 onion, sliced
- 2 garlic cloves, crushed
- 2 red or orange peppers, deseeded & sliced
- 120ml/½ cup hot chicken stock
- Low cal cooking oil spray
- Salt & pepper to taste

Method

1 Turn the slow cooker on so that it starts heating up.

2 Finely chop the pineapple & chilli and combine with the chopped coriander and soy sauce to make a salsa.

3 Place the chicken breasts in a plastic bag with the flour and give it a good shake until well coated.

4 Meanwhile place a non-stick frying pan on a low heat and gently sauté the onions, garlic & peppers in a little low cal spray for a few minutes until softened.

5 Tip the onions and peppers out of the pan onto a plate.

6 Add some more oil to the pan, increase the heat and quickly brown the chicken breasts for a minute or two to seal the meat.

7 Put the onions, peppers and chicken in the slow cooker along with the stock and combine well.

8 Load the salsa over the top of the chicken cover with the lid and leave to cook on low for 5-6 hours or high for 3-4 hours. Keep the reserved pineapple juice to hand and add a little of this during cooking if you feel the dish needs it.

9 Make sure the chicken is cooked through. Season and serve.

SERVES 4

BEGINNERS CHICKEN CURRY

260 calories per serving

······ *Ingredients* ······

- 2 onions, sliced
- 1 garlic clove, crushed
- 600g/1lb 5oz chicken breasts, cubed
- 2 tbsp tomato puree
- ½ tsp each ginger, cumin, coriander, turmeric & chilli powder

- 1 tin chopped tomatoes (400g/14oz)
- 2 tbsp fat free Greek yogurt
- Low cal cooking oil spray
- Salt & pepper to taste

······ *Method* ······

1 Turn the slow cooker on so that it starts heating up.

2 Place a non-stick frying pan on a low heat and gently sauté the onions & garlic in a little low cal spray for a few minutes until softened.

3 Put everything, except the yogurt, in the slow cooker. Combine well, cover with the lid and leave to cook on low for 5-6 hours or high for 3-4 hours.

4 Make sure the chicken is cooked through. Stir through the yogurt, season and serve.

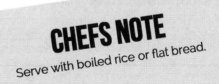

CHEFS NOTE
Serve with boiled rice or flat bread.

19

SOY & HONEY CHICKEN

300 calories per serving

Ingredients

- 4 chicken breasts, each weighing 150g/5oz
- 1 tbsp plain flour
- 1 onion, sliced
- 2 garlic cloves, crushed
- 1 tbsp honey
- 4 tbsp soy sauce
- 2 tbsp tomato puree
- 250g/1 cup fresh orange juice
- 3 medium carrots (400g/14oz), peeled & sliced into batons
- 4 handfuls spinach (200g/7oz)
- Low cal cooking oil spray
- Salt & pepper to taste

Method

1 Turn the slow cooker on so that it starts heating up.

2 Place the chicken in a plastic bag with the flour and give it a good shake until well coated.

3 Meanwhile place a non-stick frying pan on a low heat and gently sauté the onions & garlic in a little low cal spray for a few minutes until softened.

4 Tip the onions out onto a plate. Add some more oil to the pan, increase the heat and quickly brown the chicken pieces for a minute or two to seal the meat.

5 Add everything, except the spinach, to the slow cooker. Combine well, cover with the lid and leave to cook on low for 5-6 hours or high for 3-4 hours.

6 Make sure the chicken is cooked through, stir through the spinach and leave for a minute or two to gently wilt. Season and serve.

CHEFS NOTE
Serve just as it is or bulk it up with some boiled rice.

CHICKEN & SQUASH STEW

395
calories per serving

Ingredients

- 600g/1lb 5oz chicken breasts, cubed
- 1 tbsp plain flour
- 1 onion, sliced
- 2 garlic cloves, crushed
- 1 butternut squash (700g/1lb 9oz), peeled & deseeded
- 250g/1 cup hot chicken stock
- ½ tsp dried sage or thyme
- 2 tbsp low fat crème fraiche
- Low cal cooking oil spray
- Salt & pepper to taste

Method

1 Turn the slow cooker on so that it starts heating up.

2 Place the chicken in a plastic bag with the flour and give it a good shake until well coated.

3 Meanwhile place a non-stick frying pan on a low heat and gently sauté the onions & garlic in a little low cal spray for a few minutes until softened.

4 Tip the onions out onto a plate. Add some more oil to the pan, increase the heat and quickly brown the chicken pieces for a minute or two to seal the meat.

5 Cut the squash into 2cm/1 inch cubes and add everything, except the crème fraiche, to the slow cooker. Combine well, cover with the lid and leave to cook on low for 5-6 hours or high for 3-4 hours (add a little more stock if needed during cooking).

6 Make sure the chicken is cooked through and the squash is tender. Stir in the crème fraiche and leave for a minute or two to gently warm through. Season and serve.

CHEFS NOTE

This is lovely served with a portion of hot couscous.

PESTO & PEA CHICKEN

340 calories per serving

Ingredients

EASY PREP!

- 600g/1lb 5oz chicken breasts, cubed
- 2 tbsp green pesto
- 2 onions, sliced
- 120ml/½ cup hot chicken stock
- 6 handfuls frozen peas (300g/11oz)
- Low cal cooking oil spray
- Salt & pepper to taste

Method

1 Turn the slow cooker on so that it starts heating up.

2 Place the chicken in a bowl and combine with the green pesto.

3 Meanwhile place a non-stick frying pan on a low heat and gently sauté the onions & garlic in a little low cal spray for a few minutes until softened.

4 Put everything in the slow cooker. Combine well, cover with the lid and leave to cook on low for 5-6 hours or high for 3-4 hours. (add more stock if you need to)

5 Make sure the chicken is cooked through. Season and serve.

CHEFS NOTE
Throw some pre-cooked express rice into the slow cooker for the last half hour of cooking if you like.

CHICKEN & BEANS

430 calories per serving

Ingredients

- 600g/1lb 5oz chicken breasts, cubed
- 1 tbsp plain flour
- 1 onion, sliced
- 2 garlic cloves, crushed
- 1 red pepper, deseeded & sliced
- 1 tsp dried mixed herbs
- 250ml/1 cup hot chicken stock
- 2 tins cannellini beans (800g/1¾lb), drained and rinsed
- Low cal cooking oil spray
- Salt & pepper to taste

Method

1 Turn the slow cooker on so that it starts heating up.

2 Place the chicken in a plastic bag with the flour and give it a good shake until well coated.

3 Meanwhile place a non-stick frying pan on a low heat and gently sauté the onions, garlic & peppers in a little low cal spray for a few minutes until softened.

4 Tip the onions and peppers out of the pan onto a plate.

5 Add some more oil to the pan, increase the heat and quickly brown the chicken pieces for a minute or two to seal the meat.

6 Put everything in the slow cooker. Combine well, cover with the lid and leave to cook on low for 5-6 hours or high for 3-4 hours.

7 Make sure the chicken is cooked through. Season and serve.

CHEFS NOTE
Any type of tinned bean will work fine for this recipe (not baked beans though)!

HOT PULLED CHICKEN 'BURGER'

440 calories per serving

Ingredients

- 4 chicken breasts, each weighing 150g/5oz
- 5 tbsp tomato ketchup or BBQ sauce
- 250ml/1 cup hot chicken stock
- 1 tsp each ground cumin, paprika & garlic
- ½ tsp each salt & brown sugar
- 2 onions, sliced
- 4 wholemeal rolls
- Salt & pepper to taste

Method

1 Turn the slow cooker on so that it starts heating up.

2 Combine the ketchup, stock, spices, salt & sugar together to make a sauce.

3 Lay the onions over the base of the slow cooker. Sit the chicken breasts on the onions and pour the sauce over the top.

4 Put everything in the slow cooker. Combine well, cover with the lid and leave to cook on low for about 4-6 hours or until the chicken is cooked through and super tender.

5 Remove the chicken breasts and shred on a chopping board with a couple of forks. Throw the shredded chicken back into the slow cooker and combine with the sauce and onions in the bottom.

6 Leave to cook for a little longer with the lid off if the sauce is not thick enough; otherwise lay out the burger rolls and load the saucy chicken & onions straight in. Messy but delicious!!

CHEFS NOTE

Use a shop bought taco or fajita mix if you don't have the spices listed above.

CHICKEN & BACON STEW

440 calories per serving

Ingredients

- 600g/1lb 5oz chicken breasts, cubed
- 1 tbsp plain flour
- 1 onion, sliced
- 2 garlic cloves, crushed
- 4 slices lean, back bacon
- 3 handfuls new potatoes (500g/1lb 2oz), sliced
- 2 handfuls green beans (200g/7oz), chopped
- 250ml/1 cup hot chicken stock
- Low cal cooking oil spray
- Salt & pepper to taste

Method

1 Turn the slow cooker on so that it starts heating up.

2 Place the chicken in a plastic bag with the flour and give it a good shake until well coated.

3 Meanwhile place a non-stick frying pan on a low heat and gently sauté the onions, garlic & bacon in a little low cal spray for a few minutes until softened.

4 Tip the onions and bacon out of the pan onto a plate and finely chop up the bacon slices.

5 Add some more oil to the pan, increase the heat and quickly brown the chicken pieces for a minute or two to seal the meat.

6 Put everything in the slow cooker. Combine well, cover with the lid and leave to cook on low for 5-6 hours or high for 3-4 hours.

7 Make sure the chicken is cooked through and the potatoes are tender.

8 Check the seasoning and serve.

CHEFS NOTE
Cook for a little longer on high with the lid off if you need to thicken the stew up.

SPICY PEANUT BUTTER CHICKEN

330 calories per serving

Ingredients

- 2 garlic cloves, crushed
- 1 onion, sliced
- 1 tsp freshly grated ginger
- 600g/1lb 5oz chicken breasts, cubed
- 4 tbsp low fat smooth peanut butter
- ½ tsp crushed dried chillies
- 120ml/½ cup hot chicken stock
- Low cal cooking oil spray
- Salt & pepper to taste

Method

1 Turn the slow cooker on so that it starts heating up.

2 Place a large non-stick frying pan on a low heat and gently sauté the garlic, onion & ginger in a little low cal spray for a few minutes until softened (add a splash of water to the pan if you need to loosen it up).

3 Tip the softened onions onto a plate.

4 Add some more oil to the pan, increase the heat and quickly brown the chicken pieces for a minute or two to seal the meat.

5 Put everything in the slow cooker. Combine well, cover with the lid and leave to cook on low for 5-6 hours or high for 3-4 hours.

6 Make sure the chicken is cooked through. Season and serve.

CHEFS NOTE
This is good served with buttered corn-on-the-cob and steamed kale.

CHICKEN IN THICK MUSHROOM SAUCE

325 calories per serving

Ingredients

- 4 chicken breasts, each weighing 175g/6oz
- 1 leek, sliced
- 2 garlic cloves, crushed
- 1 punnet mushrooms (300g/11oz), sliced
- 1 tin low fat condensed mushroom soup (300g/11oz)

- 1 tsp mixed dried herbs
- 250ml/1 cup hot chicken stock
- Low cal cooking oil spray
- Salt & pepper to taste

Method

1 Turn the slow cooker on so that it starts heating up.

2 Place a large non-stick frying pan on a low heat and gently sauté the leek, garlic & mushrooms in a little low cal spray for a few minutes until softened (add a splash of water to the pan if you need to loosen it up).

3 Tip the softened mushrooms and leeks onto a plate.

4 Add some more oil to the pan, increase the heat and quickly brown the chicken breasts for a minute or two to seal the meat.

5 Put everything in the slow cooker. Combine well, cover with the lid and leave to cook on low for 5-6 hours or high for 3-4 hours.

6 Make sure the chicken is cooked through. Season and serve.

CHEFS NOTE
Try serving with a mound of shredded steamed cabbage.

27

CREAMY MUSTARD CHICKEN

385 calories per serving

Ingredients

- 4 chicken breasts, each weighing 175g/6oz
- 1 onion, sliced
- 1 garlic clove, crushed
- 2 tbsp Dijon mustard
- 2 handfuls green beans (200g/7oz), sliced
- 120ml/½ cup hot chicken stock
- 4 tbsp low fat crème fraiche
- Low cal cooking oil spray
- Salt & pepper to taste

Method

1 Turn the slow cooker on so that it starts heating up.

2 Place a large non-stick frying pan on a low heat and gently sauté the onion & garlic in a little low cal spray for a few minutes until softened.

3 Tip the softened onions onto a plate.

4 Add some more oil to the pan, increase the heat and quickly brown the chicken breasts for a minute or two to seal the meat.

5 Put everything, except the crème fraiche in the slow cooker. Combine well, cover with the lid and leave to cook on high for 3-4 hours (add a little more stock during cooking if needed).

6 Make sure the chicken is cooked through. Stir through the creme fraiche and leave to warm for a minute or two.

7 Check the seasoning and serve.

CHEFS NOTE

This recipe is great served with a fluffy baked potato or on a bed of fresh spinach.

CRUST-LESS CHICKEN & HAM PIE

280 calories per serving

Ingredients

- 500g/1lb 2oz chicken breasts, cubed
- 5 slices cooked ham, chopped
- 2 tbsp plain flour
- 1 tbsp low fat 'butter' spread
- 250ml/1 cup hot chicken stock
- 1 onion, sliced
- ½ tsp mixed dried herbs
- Low cal cooking oil spray
- Salt & pepper to taste

Method

1 Turn the slow cooker on so that it starts heating up.

2 Gently heat a saucepan on a low heat and melt the 'butter'. Using a wooden spoon stir through the flour to make a roux (paste). When you have a paste start adding the hot stock and, using a hand whisk, gently beat until you end up with a smooth sauce.

3 Place everything into the slow cooker combine well, cover with the lid and leave to cook on low for 5-6 hours or high for 3-4 hours.

4 Make sure the chicken is cooked through. Check the seasoning and serve.

CHEFS NOTE
This traditional pie filling is lovely served with creamy mashed potatoes and/or steamed spring greens.

SPICED CHICKEN & SULTANAS

360 calories per serving

Ingredients

- 1 red onion, sliced
- 1 garlic clove, crushed
- 600g/1lb 5oz chicken breasts, cubed
- 3 tbsp tomato puree
- 120ml/½ cup hot chicken stock
- 1 tbsp mild curry powder
- 2 medium carrots (250g/9oz), cut into batons

- 4 tbsp sultanas, chopped
- 1 tbsp ground almonds
- 3 tbsp fat free Greek yogurt
- Low cal cooking oil spray
- Salt & pepper to taste

Method

1 Turn the slow cooker on so that it starts heating up.

2 Place a non-stick frying pan on a low heat and gently sauté the onions & garlic in a little low cal spray for a few minutes until softened.

3 Put everything in the slow cooker, except the yogurt. Combine well, cover with the lid and leave to cook on low for 5-6 hours or high for 3-4 hours (add a little more stock during cooking if you need to).

4 Make sure the chicken is cooked through. Stir through the yogurt, season and serve.

CHEFS NOTE
Serve with boiled rice and some fresh chopped almonds if you wish.

CHICKEN & ROSEMARY STEW

310 calories per serving

Ingredients

- 4 chicken breasts, each weighing 175g/6oz
- 1 onion, sliced
- 2 garlic cloves, crushed
- 2 tbsp tomato puree
- 60ml/¼ cup hot chicken stock
- 1 tbsp Worcestershire sauce
- 1 tbsp freshly chopped rosemary (or 2 tsp dried rosemary is fine)
- 2 tins chopped tomatoes (800g/1¾lb)
- Low cal cooking oil spray
- Salt & pepper to taste

Method

1 Turn the slow cooker on so that it starts heating up.

2 Meanwhile place a non-stick frying pan on a low heat and gently sauté the onions & garlic in a little low cal spray for a few minutes until softened.

3 Put everything in the slow cooker. Combine well, cover with the lid and leave to cook on low for 5-6 hours or high for 3-4 hours (add a little more stock during cooking if needed).

4 Make sure the chicken is cooked through, season and serve.

CHEFS NOTE
Keep this dish nice and light by serving with a fresh watercress salad.

WINTER STEW

385
calories per serving

Ingredients

- 600g/1lb 5oz chicken breasts, thickly sliced
- 1 onion, sliced
- 2 garlic cloves, crushed
- 250ml/1 cup hot chicken stock
- 1 medium potato (200g/7oz), peeled & grated
- 2 medium parsnips (200g/7oz), peeled & grated
- 2 medium carrots (250g/9oz), peeled & sliced
- 1 tbsp freshly chopped thyme
- Low cal cooking oil spray
- Salt & pepper to taste

Method

1 Turn the slow cooker on so that it starts heating up.

2 Meanwhile place a non-stick frying pan on a low heat and gently sauté the onions & garlic in a little low cal spray for a few minutes until softened.

3 Put everything in the slow cooker. Combine well, cover with the lid and leave to cook on low for 5-6 hours or high for 3-4 hours (add a little more stock during cooking if needed).

4 Make sure the chicken is cooked through, season and serve.

CHEFS NOTE
Use dried thyme if you don't have fresh thyme to hand.

GREEN THAI CHICKEN

375
calories per serving

Ingredients

- 2 onions, sliced
- 1 garlic clove, crushed
- 600g/1lb 5oz chicken breasts, cubed
- 1 tbsp Thai green curry paste
- 1 tbsp coconut cream
- 250ml/1 cup hot chicken stock
- 4 handfuls frozen peas (200g/7oz)
- 2 tbsp fat free Greek yogurt
- Low cal cooking oil spray
- Salt & pepper to taste

Method

1 Turn the slow cooker on so that it starts heating up.

2 Place a non-stick frying pan on a low heat and gently sauté the onions & garlic in a little low cal spray for a few minutes until softened.

3 Put everything, except the yogurt, in the slow cooker. Combine well, cover with the lid and leave to cook on low for 5-6 hours or high for 3-4 hours.

4 Make sure the chicken is cooked through. Stir through the yogurt, season and serve.

CHEFS NOTE
Serve with rice or noodles and lime wedges.

SWEET CHILLI CHICKEN

280 calories per serving

Ingredients

- 2 onions, sliced
- 1 garlic clove, crushed
- 600g/1lb 5oz chicken breasts, cubed
- 2 tbsp honey
- ½ red chilli, deseeded & finely chopped
- 2 tsp cornflour, dissolved in a little warm water

- 120ml/½ cup chicken stock
- 2 handfuls green beans (200g/7oz), chopped
- Low cal cooking oil spray
- Salt & pepper to taste

Method

1 Turn the slow cooker on so that it starts heating up.

2 Place a non-stick frying pan on a low heat and gently sauté the onions & garlic in a little low cal spray for a few minutes until softened.

3 Put everything in the slow cooker. Combine well, cover with the lid and leave to cook on low for 5-6 hours or high for 3-4 hours (add some more stock during cooking of needed).

4 Make sure the chicken is cooked through. Season and serve.

CHEFS NOTE
Add the green beans much later during cooking if you prefer them crunchy.

MEXICAN SHREDDED CHICKEN

305
calories per serving

Ingredients

- 4 chicken breasts, each weighing 175g/6oz
- 1 onion, sliced
- 2 garlic cloves, crushed
- 1 tsp chipotle paste
- 1 tin chopped tomatoes (400g/14oz)
- ½ tsp brown sugar
- 120ml/½ cup hot chicken stock
- 1 red onion
- 2 tbsp freshly chopped coriander
- Low cal cooking oil spray
- Salt & pepper to taste

Method

1 Turn the slow cooker on so that it starts heating up and season the chicken breasts.

2 Place a non-stick frying pan on a low heat and gently sauté the onions & garlic in a little low cal spray for a few minutes until softened.

3 Stir through the chipotle paste, chopped tomatoes, sugar & stock for a minute or two.

4 Add everything, except the red onion and fresh coriander, to the slow cooker. Combine well, cover with the lid and leave to cook on low for 5-6 hours or high for 3-4 hours (add a little more stock during cooking if needed).

5 When the chicken breasts are tender remove the meat and place on a shopping board. Use two forks to finely shred each breast and then return the meat to the slow cooker. Combine well.

6 While this continues to cook prepare the red onion by peeling and slicing into very thin rings.

7 Serve the chicken in shallow bowls topped with raw onion rings and chopped coriander.

CHEFS NOTE

Use Tabasco sauce or any other hot chilli sauce if you don't have chipotle paste.

SWEET CHICKEN LINGUINE

470 calories per serving

Ingredients

- 4 chicken breasts, each weighing 125g/4oz
- 1 onion
- 1 garlic clove, crushed
- 2 tsp honey
- 120ml/½ cup hot chicken stock

- ½ lemon, thinly sliced
- 2 handfuls tenderstem broccoli (200g/7oz), roughly chopped
- 300g/11oz dried linguine pasta
- Salt & pepper to taste

Method

1 Turn the slow cooker on so that it starts heating up and season the chicken breasts.

2 Add everything, except the broccoli and linguine, to the slow cooker. Combine well, cover with the lid and leave to cook on low for 5-6 hours or high for 3-4 hours (add a little more stock during cooking if needed).

3 When the chicken breasts are tender remove the meat and place on a shopping board. Use two forks to finely shred each breast and then return the meat to the slow cooker. Combine well.

4 Meanwhile cook the linguine in a pan of salted boiling water until tender. Add the broccoli for the last 2 minutes of cooking.

5 Pick the lemon slices out of the slow cooker. Drain the pasta & broccoli and toss in with the sweet shredded chicken.

6 Season and serve.

CHEFS NOTE
Serve with some fresh chopped herbs if you have any to hand.

BBQ CHICKEN DRUMMERS

195 calories per serving

Ingredients

- 8 skinless chicken drumsticks, each weighing about 125g/4oz
- 1 tbsp honey
- 3 tbsp soy sauce
- 1 tsp paprika
- 2 garlic cloves, crushed
- Salt & pepper to taste

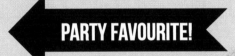
PARTY FAVOURITE!

Method

1 Turn the slow cooker on so that it starts heating up (don't do this if you are marinating the chicken overnight).

2 Stab each of the chicken drumsticks a few times with a fork to penetrate the meat.

3 Mix together the honey, soy sauce, paprika & garlic to make a marinade.

4 Smother the drumsticks in the marinade, place in a bowl and leave to marinade for as long as possible (overnight if you can).

5 Place in the slow cooker, cover with the lid and leave to cook on high for 2-4 hours or until the chicken is cooked through.

CHEFS NOTE
Serves 4 as part of a BBQ or 2 as a main course.

SLOW COOKED CHICKEN WINGS

370 calories per serving

Ingredients

- 16 skinless chicken wings, each about weighing 75g/3oz
- 2 tsp garlic powder
- 2 tsp paprika
- 1 tsp cumin powder
- ½ tsp each salt & sugar
- 4 tbsp Worcestershire sauce
- Salt & pepper to taste

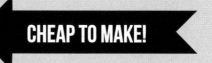

CHEAP TO MAKE!

Method

1 Turn the slow cooker on so that it starts heating up (don't do this if you are marinating the chicken overnight).

2 Stab each of the chicken wings a few times with a fork to penetrate the meat.

3 Mix together the garlic, paprika, cumin, salt, sugar & Worcestershire sauce to make a marinade (make up more if you need to).

4 Smother the in the marinade, place in a bowl and leave to marinade for as long as possible (overnight if you can).

5 Place in the slow cooker, cover with the lid and leave to cook on high for 2-4 hours or until the chicken is cooked through.

CHEFS NOTE
Serves 4 as part of a BBQ or 2 as a main course.

CASHEW CHICKEN STEW

410 calories per serving

Ingredients

- 4 chicken breasts, each weighing 175g/6oz
- 1 tbsp plain flour
- 1 onion, sliced
- 2 garlic cloves, crushed
- 1 tbsp freshly grated ginger
- 2 red or orange peppers, deseeded & sliced
- 1 tbsp tomato puree
- 120ml/½ cup hot chicken stock
- 1 handful (75g/3oz) cashew nuts
- Low cal cooking oil spray
- Salt & pepper to taste

Method

1 Turn the slow cooker on so that it starts heating up.

2 Place the chicken in a plastic bag with the flour and give it a good shake until well coated.

3 Meanwhile place a non-stick frying pan on a low heat and gently sauté the onions, garlic, ginger & peppers in a little low cal spray for a few minutes until softened.

4 Tip the onions and peppers out of the pan onto a plate.

5 Add some more oil to the pan, increase the heat and quickly brown the chicken pieces for a minute or two to seal the meat.

6 Put everything in the slow cooker. Combine well, cover with the lid and leave to cook on low for 5-6 hours or high for 3-4 hours (add a little more stock during cooking if you need to).

7 Make sure the chicken is cooked through. Thickly slice the chicken breasts, season and serve.

CHEFS NOTE

Serve with noodles or a simple watercress salad.

ROSEMARY CHICKEN BUTTER BEANS

SERVES 4

490 calories per serving

Ingredients

- 600g/1lb 5oz chicken breasts, cubed
- 1 tbsp plain flour
- 2 tsp dried rosemary
- 1 onion, sliced
- 2 garlic cloves, crushed
- 250ml/1 cup hot chicken stock
- 2 tins butter beans (800g/1¾lb), drained and rinsed
- 1 lime, cut into wedges
- Low cal cooking oil spray
- Salt & pepper to taste

Method

1 Turn the slow cooker on so that it starts heating up.

2 Place the chicken in a plastic bag with the flour & dried rosemary and give it a good shake until well coated.

3 Meanwhile place a non-stick frying pan on a low heat and gently sauté the onions & garlic in a little low cal spray for a few minutes until softened.

4 Tip the onions out of the pan onto a plate.

5 Add some more oil to the pan, increase the heat and quickly brown the chicken for a minute or two to seal the meat.

6 Put everything in the slow cooker. Combine well, cover with the lid and leave to cook on low for 5-6 hours or high for 3-4 hours.

7 Make sure the chicken is cooked through. Season and serve with the lime wedges.

CHEFS NOTE
The fresh taste of the lime wedges really lifts this meal when serving.

ZUCCHINI & CHICKEN STEW

305 calories per serving

Ingredients

- 4 chicken breasts, each weighing 175g/6oz
- 1 onion, sliced
- 2 garlic cloves, crushed
- 4 tbsp freshly chopped basil (reserve a little for garnish)
- 120ml/½ cup hot chicken stock
- 1 tin chopped tomatoes (400g/14oz)
- 4 medium courgettes (400g/14oz), sliced lengthways
- 1 tbsp grated Parmesan cheese
- Low cal cooking oil spray
- Salt & pepper to taste

Method

1 Turn the slow cooker on so that it starts heating up.

2 Place a non-stick frying pan on a low heat and gently sauté the onions & garlic in a little low cal spray for a few minutes until softened.

3 Put everything, except the Parmesan cheese, in the slow cooker. Combine well, cover with the lid and leave to cook on low for 5-6 hours or high for 3-4 hours.

4 Make sure the chicken is cooked through, sprinkle with the grated Parmesan & reserved fresh basil and serve.

CHEFS NOTE
Use dried basil or mixed herbs if you don't have fresh basil and try serving with creamy mashed potatoes.

SPANISH RICE STEW

495 calories per serving

Ingredients

- 500g/1lb 2oz chicken breasts, cubed
- 1 onion, sliced
- ½ red chilli, deseeded & finely sliced
- 1-2 small chorizo sausages (75g/3oz), finely chopped
- 2 garlic cloves, crushed
- 200g/7oz rice
- 500ml/2 cups hot chicken stock
- ½ tin chopped tomatoes (200g/7oz)
- 2 handfuls frozen peas (100g/3½oz)
- 1 tsp paprika
- Low cal cooking oil spray
- Salt & pepper to taste

Method

1 Turn the slow cooker on so that it starts heating up.

2 Place a non-stick frying pan on a low heat and gently sauté the onions, chilli, chopped chorizo & garlic in a little low cal spray for a few minutes until softened.

3 Tip the onions and chorizo out of the pan onto a plate.

4 Add some more oil, increase the heat and quickly brown the chicken pieces for a minute or two to seal the meat.

5 Put everything in the slow cooker. Combine well, cover with the lid and leave to cook on low for 5-6 hours or high for 3-4 hours (add a little more stock during cooking if needed).

6 Make sure the chicken is cooked through and the rice is tender.

7 Check the seasoning and serve.

CHEFS NOTE
Chorizo is a classic Spanish meat but it's fine to use any spicy salami you like.

CHERRY TOMATO & COCONUT MILK CHICKEN

315
calories per serving

Ingredients

- 500g/1lb 2oz chicken breasts, cubed
- 1 onion, sliced
- 2 garlic cloves, crushed
- ½ red chilli, deseeded & finely sliced
- 1 punnet ripe cherry tomatoes (300g/11oz), quartered
- 1 tsp turmeric
- 120ml/½ cup low fat coconut milk
- 2 tbsp tomato puree
- 4 handfuls spinach (200g/7oz)
- Low cal cooking oil spray
- Salt & pepper to taste

Method

1 Turn the slow cooker on so that it starts heating up.

2 Place a large non-stick frying pan on a low heat and gently sauté the onions, garlic, chilli & cherry tomatoes in a little low cal spray for 5-10 minutes or until softened.

3 Put everything in the slow cooker. Combine well, cover with the lid and leave to cook on low for 5-6 hours or high for 3-4 hours (add a little more coconut milk or chicken stock during cooking if needed).

4 Make sure the chicken is cooked through. Check the seasoning and serve.

CHEFS NOTE
Try not adding the spinach until the very end so that it still has a crunch to it.

WHITE WINE & CHICKEN STEW

SERVES 4

385 calories per serving

Ingredients

- 1 onion, sliced
- 3 garlic cloves, crushed
- 2 tbsp plain flour
- 1 tbsp low fat 'butter' spread
- 120ml/½ cup hot chicken stock
- 120ml/½ cup white wine

- 500g/1lb 2oz chicken breasts, cubed
- 2 medium carrots (300g/11oz), finely chopped
- 1 punnet mushrooms (300g/11oz), sliced
- Low cal cooking oil spray
- Salt & pepper to taste

Method

1 Turn the slow cooker on so that it starts heating up.

2 Place a non-stick frying pan on a low heat and gently sauté the onions & garlic in a little low cal spray for a few minutes until softened.

3 Mix the wine and hot stock together in a cup.

4 Gently heat a saucepan on a low heat and melt the 'butter'. Using a wooden spoon stir through the flour to make a roux (paste). When you have a paste start adding the hot stock/wine and, using a hand whisk, gently whisk until you end up with a smooth sauce.

5 Place everything into the slow cooker combine well, cover with the lid and leave to cook on low for 5-6 hours or high for 3-4 hours (add a little more stock during cooking if needed).

6 Make sure the chicken is cooked through and the carrots are tender. Check the seasoning and serve.

CHEFS NOTE
Garnish with lots of freshly ground black pepper and chopped flat leaf parsley if you have it.

MOROCCAN STEW

495
calories per
serving

Ingredients

- 1 onion, sliced
- 2 garlic cloves, crushed
- 400g/14oz chicken breasts, cubed
- 1 tsp each turmeric & cumin
- 1 cinnamon stick
- ½ tin chickpeas (200g/7oz), drained

- 6 dried apricots, finely chopped
- 200g/7oz rice
- 500ml/2 cups hot chicken stock
- ½ tin chopped tomatoes (200g/7oz)
- Low cal cooking oil spray
- Salt & pepper to taste

Method

1 Turn the slow cooker on so that it starts heating up.

2 Place a non-stick frying pan on a low heat and gently sauté the onions & garlic in a little low cal spray for a few minutes until softened.

3 Tip the onions out of the pan onto a plate.

4 Add some more oil, increase the heat and quickly brown the chicken pieces for a minute or two to seal the meat.

5 Put everything in the slow cooker. Combine well, cover with the lid and leave to cook on low for 5-6 hours or high for 3-4 hours (add a little more stock during cooking if needed).

6 Make sure the chicken is cooked through and the rice is tender.

7 Remove the cinamon stick. Check the seasoning and serve.

CHEFS NOTE
Use sultanas in place of apricots and try some freshly chopped coriander too.

Skinny
SLOW COOKER
Student
MEAT DISHES

MOREISH MEATBALLS

390
calories per
serving

Ingredients

- 1 onion, sliced
- 1 garlic clove, crushed
- 600g/1lb 5oz lean minced beef
- 2 tbsp breadcrumbs
- 1 carrot (150g/4oz), grated
- 1 tsp ground cumin

- 1 egg
- 2 tbsp tomato puree
- 500ml/2 cups tomato passata
- ½ tsp each salt & brown sugar
- Low cal cooking oil spray
- Salt & pepper to taste

Method

1 Turn the slow cooker on so that it starts heating up.

2 Place a non-stick frying pan on a low heat and gently sauté the onions & garlic in a little low cal spray for a few minutes until softened.

3 Meanwhile make breadcrumbs by taking the end crust from a loaf of bread and grate. Combine together the beef, breadcrumbs, carrot, cumin & egg (use a mixer to do this if you've got one, just use your hands if not).

4 Once everything is well combined shape into about 20 small firm meatballs.

5 Add everything to the slow cooker. Combine well, cover with the lid and leave to cook on low for 5-6 hours or high for 3-4 hours (give the meatballs a stir once or twice during cooking to keep them covered in sauce).

6 Check the seasoning of the sauce and serve.

CHEFS NOTE
Serve with spaghetti, rice or flat bread.

CREAMY BEEF STEW

375
calories per serving

Ingredients

- 600g/1lb 5oz lean stewing beef
- 1 tbsp plain flour
- 1 onion, sliced
- 1 red pepper, deseeded & sliced
- 2 garlic cloves, crushed
- 2 tins chopped tomatoes (800g/1¾lb)
- 2 tsp paprika
- 60ml/¼ cup beef stock
- 3 tbsp tomato puree
- 2 tbsp fat free Greek yogurt
- Low cal cooking oil spray
- Salt & pepper to taste

Method

1 Turn the slow cooker on so that it starts heating up.

2 Place the beef in a plastic bag with the flour and give it a good shake until well coated.

3 Meanwhile place a non-stick frying pan on a low heat and gently sauté the onions, garlic & peppers in a little low cal spray for a few minutes until softened.

4 Tip the onions and peppers out of the pan onto a plate.

5 Add some more oil to the pan, increase the heat and quickly brown the beef pieces for a minute or two to seal the meat.

6 Add everything, except the yogurt, to the slow cooker. Combine well, cover with the lid and leave to cook on low for 5-6 hours or until the beef is meltingly tender (add a little more stock if you need to during cooking)

7 When the stew is cooked through, stir through the yogurt and serve.

CHEFS NOTE
Serve with rice or potatoes, or load some halved new potatoes and chunky carrots into the slow cooker at the beginning.

SERVES 4

LAMB & BUTTER BEAN STEW

400 calories per serving

Ingredients

- 600g/1lb 5oz lean lamb leg or shoulder, cubed
- 1 tbsp plain flour
- 1 onion, sliced
- 2 garlic cloves, crushed
- 250ml/1 cup chicken stock
- 1 tin butter beans (400g/14oz), drained & rinsed
- 3 handfuls spinach (150g/5oz)
- ½ tsp each paprika, cumin & coriander
- ½ tsp ground ginger
- Low cal cooking oil spray
- Salt & pepper to taste

Method

1 Turn the slow cooker on so that it starts heating up.

2 Place the lamb in a plastic bag with the flour and give it a good shake until well coated.

3 Meanwhile place a non-stick frying pan on a low heat and gently sauté the onions & garlic in a little low cal spray for a few minutes until softened.

4 Tip the onions out of the pan onto a plate.

5 Add some more oil to the pan, increase the heat and quickly brown the lamb for a minute or two to seal the meat.

6 Add everything to the slow cooker. Combine well, cover with the lid and leave to cook on low for 5-6 hours or until the lamb is tender (add a little more stock if you need to during cooking)

7 When the stew is cooked through, check the seasoning and serve.

CHEFS NOTE
If you prefer you can add the spinach at the very end of cooking to give the stew a fresh taste.

BEEF & PEA KEEMA

345 calories per serving

Ingredients

- 1 onion, sliced
- 1 garlic clove, crushed
- 600g/1lb 5oz lean minced beef
- 1 tsp each ground cumin, turmeric & coriander
- ½ tsp chilli powder

- 1 tin chopped tomatoes (400g/14oz)
- 3 tbsp tomato puree
- 4 handfuls frozen peas (200g/7oz)
- Low cal cooking oil spray
- Salt & pepper to taste

Method

1 Turn the slow cooker on so that it starts heating up.

2 Place a non-stick frying pan on a low heat and gently sauté the onions & garlic in a little low cal spray for a few minutes until softened.

3 Tip the onions out of the pan onto a plate.

4 Add some more oil to the pan, increase the heat and quickly brown the mince for a minute or two.

5 Add everything to the slow cooker. Combine well, cover with the lid and leave to cook on low for 5-6 hours or high for 3-4 hours.

6 Check the seasoning of the sauce and serve.

CHEFS NOTE
Use a tablespoon of curry powder if you don't have the single spices listed.

THREE BEAN BEEF CHILLI

430 calories per serving

Ingredients

- 1 red onion, sliced
- 1 garlic clove, crushed
- 1 red pepper, deseeded & sliced
- 1 carrot (150g/5oz), peeled & finely diced
- 600g/1lb 5oz lean minced beef
- 1 tsp each ground cumin & turmeric
- 2 red chillies, deseeded & finely chopped
- 1 tin mixed beans (400g/14oz), drained & rinsed
- 250ml/1 cup tomato pasatta
- 3 tbsp tomato puree
- Low cal cooking oil spray
- Salt & pepper to taste

Method

1 Turn the slow cooker on so that it starts heating up.

2 Place a non-stick frying pan on a low heat and gently sauté the onions, garlic, peppers & carrots in a little low cal spray for a few minutes until softened.

3 Tip the onions, peppers & carrots out of the pan onto a plate.

4 Add some more oil to the pan, increase the heat and quickly brown the mince for a minute or two.

5 Add everything to the slow cooker. Combine well, cover with the lid and leave to cook on low for 5-6 hours or high for 3-4 hours.

6 Check the seasoning of the sauce and serve.

CHEFS NOTE
Add a little more beef stock to the slow cooker if you need to during cooking.

MEXICAN BLACK EYE STEW

430 calories per serving

Ingredients

- 1 onion, sliced
- 2 garlic cloves, crushed
- 600g/1lb 5oz lean minced beef
- 1 tsp each chilli powder, paprika, cumin & oregano
- 1 tin black eye beans (400g/14oz), drained & rinsed

- 1 tin chopped tomatoes (400g/14oz)
- 2 tbsp tomato puree
- 1 red onion
- Low cal cooking oil spray
- Salt & pepper to taste

Method

1 Turn the slow cooker on so that it starts heating up.

2 Place a non-stick frying pan on a low heat and gently sauté the onions & garlic in a little low cal spray for a few minutes until softened.

3 Tip the onions out of the pan onto a plate.

4 Add some more oil to the pan, increase the heat and quickly brown the mince for a minute or two.

5 Add everything, except the red onion, to the slow cooker. Combine well, cover with the lid and leave to cook on low for 5-6 hours or high for 3-4 hours.

6 Peel the red onion and cut into thin rings. Use this to serve over the top of the chilli along with some rice or tortilla chips.

CHEFS NOTE
If you have any chopped fresh coriander use this as a garnish with the red onion too.

SIMPLE SPAG BOL

335
calories per
serving

Ingredients

- 1 onion, chopped
- 1 garlic clove, crushed
- 1 tbsp Worcestershire sauce or marmite
- 1 carrot (150g/5oz), peeled & finely diced
- 600g/1lb 5oz lean minced beef
- 1 tsp each ground oregano or basil
- 1 tin chopped tomatoes (400g/14oz)
- 250ml/1 cup tomato pasatta
- 3 tbsp tomato puree
- Low cal cooking oil spray
- Salt & pepper to taste

Method

1 Turn the slow cooker on so that it starts heating up.

2 Add everything to the slow cooker. Combine well, cover with the lid and leave to cook on low for 5-6 hours or high for 3-4 hours or until everything is cooked through (cook for a little longer with the lid off if you want the sauce to thicken up).

3 Check the seasoning of the sauce and serve with a pile of spaghetti.

CHEFS NOTE
No browning, no sautéing, no nothing. Just whack it all in and eat up.

LAMB & LENTILS

425
calories per
serving

Ingredients

- 500g/1lb 2oz lean lamb leg or shoulder, cubed
- 1 tbsp plain flour
- 1 celery stalk, chopped
- 1 onion, sliced
- 2 garlic cloves, crushed

- 150g/5oz red lentils
- 1 tsp dried rosemary
- 750ml/3 cups beef stock
- Low cal cooking oil spray
- Salt & pepper to taste

Method

1 Turn the slow cooker on so that it starts heating up.

2 Place the lamb in a plastic bag with the flour and give it a good shake until well coated.

3 Meanwhile place a non-stick frying pan on a low heat and gently sauté the celery, onions & garlic in a little low cal spray for a few minutes until softened.

4 Tip the onions and celery out of the pan onto a plate.

5 Add some more oil to the pan, increase the heat and quickly brown the lamb for a minute or two to seal the meat.

6 Add everything to the slow cooker. Combine well, cover with the lid and leave to cook on low for 5-6 hours or until the lamb is really tender and the lentils are cooked through (add a little more stock if you need to during cooking)

7 When the stew is ready, check the seasoning and serve.

CHEFS NOTE
This also works really well using lamb on the bone. Cook until the lamb falls away with ease.

NUTTY BEEF & ONIONS

360
calories per
serving

Ingredients

- 600g/1lb 5oz lean stewing beef, cubed
- 1 tbsp plain flour
- 3 onions, sliced
- 2 garlic cloves, crushed
- 1 tbsp ground almonds
- 250ml/1 cup beef stock
- 1 tsp paprika
- Low cal cooking oil spray
- Salt & pepper to taste

Method

1 Turn the slow cooker on so that it starts heating up.

2 Place the beef in a plastic bag with the flour and give it a good shake until well coated.

3 Meanwhile place a non-stick frying pan on a low heat and gently sauté the onions & garlic in a little low cal spray for a few minutes until softened.

4 Tip the onions out of the pan onto a plate.

5 Add some more oil to the pan, increase the heat and quickly brown the beef pieces for a minute or two to seal the meat.

6 Add everything to the slow cooker. Combine well, cover with the lid and leave to cook on low for 5-6 hours or until the beef is really tender (add a little more stock if you need to during cooking)

7 When the stew is cooked through, season and serve.

CHEFS NOTE
Try stirring a pile of fresh spinach through the stew just before serving.

SAUSAGE & BEAN CASSEROLE

395 calories per serving

Ingredients

- 6 lean pork sausages
- 1 onion, sliced
- 1 green pepper, deseeded & sliced
- 2 garlic cloves, crushed
- 1 tin chopped tomatoes (400g/14oz)
- 1 tin borlotti beans (400g/14oz), rinsed & drained

- 1 tbsp Dijon mustard
- 3 tbsp tomato puree
- 2 tsp Worcestershire sauce
- 1 tsp dried mixed herbs
- Low cal cooking oil spray
- Salt & pepper to taste

Method

1 Turn the slow cooker on so that it starts heating up.

2 Place a non-stick frying pan on a low heat and gently brown the sausages for a few minutes. Take the sausages out of the pan and slice into discs about 1cm/½ inch thick.

3 Add some more low cal oil to the pan and sauté the onions, garlic & peppers for a few minutes until softened.

4 Add everything to the slow cooker. Combine well, cover with the lid and leave to cook on low for 5-6 hours or high for 3-4 hours.

5 Check the seasoning and serve.

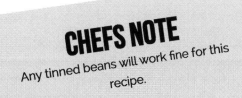

CHEFS NOTE
Any tinned beans will work fine for this recipe.

SERVES 4

SLOW BEEF CURRY

335
calories per
serving

Ingredients

- 600g/1lb 5oz lean stewing beef
- 2 onions, sliced
- 3 garlic cloves, crushed
- 2 tins chopped tomatoes (800g/1 ¾ lb)
- 1 tsp each cumin, coriander, turmeric, ginger & chilli powder
- 60ml/¼ cup beef stock
- Low cal cooking oil spray
- Salt & pepper to taste

Method

1 Turn the slow cooker on so that it starts heating up.

2 Place a non-stick frying pan on a low heat and gently sauté the onions & garlic in a little low cal spray for a few minutes until softened.

3 Tip the onions out of the pan onto a plate.

4 Add some more oil to the pan, increase the heat and quickly brown the beef for a minute or two to seal the meat.

5 Add everything to the slow cooker. Combine well, cover with the lid and leave to cook on low for 6-7 hours or until the beef is meltingly tender (add a little more stock if you need to during cooking)

6 Season and serve with rice or flat bread.

CHEFS NOTE
Try chopping some onions and combining with a couple of tablespoons of mango chutney to make a fruity side for your curry.

TENDER PORK RIBS

380
calories per serving

Ingredients

- 1.5kg/3lb 6oz pork ribs
- 1lt/4 cups chicken stock
- 2 tsp paprika
- 2 tsp brown sugar
- Salt & pepper to taste

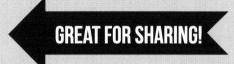

GREAT FOR SHARING!

Method

1 Turn the slow cooker on so that it starts heating up.

2 Add everything to the slow cooker. Combine well, cover with the lid and leave to cook on low for 7-9 hours or until the ribs are super tender (the ribs should be covered in liquid so add a little more stock if you need to during cooking).

3 Season and serve with BBQ sauce

CHEFS NOTE
After slow cooking try brushing the ribs in BBQ sauce and whacking in a really hot oven for 10- 15 minutes until crispy.

RED ONION & MUSHROOM BEEF STEW

370 calories per serving

Ingredients

- 600g/1lb 5oz lean stewing beef
- 1 tbsp plain flour
- 1 tsp paprika
- 2 red onions, sliced
- 2 garlic cloves, crushed

- 1 punnet mushrooms (300g/11oz), sliced
- 380ml/1½ cups hot beef stock
- Low cal cooking oil spray
- Salt & pepper to taste

Method

1 Turn the slow cooker on so that it starts heating up.

2 Place the beef in a plastic bag with the flour & paprika and give it a good shake until well coated.

3 Meanwhile place a non-stick frying pan on a low heat and gently sauté the red onions & garlic in a little low cal spray for a few minutes until softened.

4 Tip the onions out of the pan onto a plate.

5 Add some more oil to the pan, increase the heat and quickly brown the beef pieces for a minute or two to seal the meat.

6 Add everything to the slow cooker. Combine well, cover with the lid and leave to cook on low for 5-6 hours or until the beef is meltingly tender (add a little more stock if you need to during cooking)

7 When the stew is cooked through, check the seasoning and serve.

CHEFS NOTE

Try adding some shredded spring greens half an hour before the end of cooking for some fresh goodness.

CHINESE PORK STEW

345 calories per serving

Ingredients

- 600g/1lb 5oz lean pork shoulder, diced
- 1 tbsp plain flour
- 2 tsp Chinese five spice powder
- 2 tsp brown sugar
- 1 onion, sliced
- 2 garlic cloves, crushed
- 3 tbsp soy sauce
- 4 pak choi, quartered
- 370ml/1½ cups chicken stock
- Low cal cooking oil spray
- Salt & pepper to taste

Method

1 Turn the slow cooker on so that it starts heating up.

2 Place the beef in a plastic bag with the flour & five spice powder and give it a good shake until well coated.

3 Meanwhile place a non-stick frying pan on a low heat and gently sauté the onions & garlic in a little low cal spray for a few minutes until softened.

4 Tip the onions out of the pan onto a plate.

5 Add some more oil to the pan, increase the heat and quickly brown the pork pieces for a minute or two to seal the meat.

6 Add everything to the slow cooker. Combine well, cover with the lid and leave to cook on low for 5-6 hours or until the pork is really tender (add a little more stock if you need to during cooking)

7 When the stew is cooked through, check the seasoning and serve.

CHEFS NOTE

Pak choi is a widely available cabbage popular in Asian cooking. Feel free to substitute for pointed cabbage if you like.

HEARTY SIMPLE STEW

470
calories per serving

Ingredients

- 600g/1lb 5oz lean stewing beef, cubed
- 1 tbsp plain flour
- 2 onions, sliced
- 2 garlic cloves, crushed
- 3 medium carrots (400g/14oz), peeled & sliced
- 2 handfuls new potatoes (400g/14oz), halved
- 1 tsp dried thyme
- 50g/2oz pearl barley
- 500ml/2 cups beef stock
- Low cal cooking oil spray
- Salt & pepper to taste

Method

1 Turn the slow cooker on so that it starts heating up.

2 Place the beef in a plastic bag with the flour and give it a good shake until well coated.

3 Meanwhile place a non-stick frying pan on a low heat and gently sauté the onions & garlic in a little low cal spray for a few minutes until softened.

4 Tip the onions out of the pan onto a plate.

5 Add some more oil to the pan, increase the heat and quickly brown the beef pieces for a minute or two to seal the meat.

6 Add everything to the slow cooker. Combine well, cover with the lid and leave to cook on low for 5-7 hours or until the beef is meltingly tender (add a little more stock if you need to during cooking)

7 When the stew is cooked through check the seasoning and serve.

CHEFS NOTE
A handful of chopped flat leaf parsley makes a good garnish for this simple regional stew.

LAMB & SWEET POTATO

450 calories per serving

Ingredients

- 600g/1lb 5oz lean lamb leg or shoulder, cubed
- 1 onion, sliced
- 2 garlic cloves, crushed
- 3 medium (500g/1lb 2oz) sweet potato, peeled & cut into chunks
- 1 tin (400g/14oz) tinned chopped tomatoes

- 1 tsp each ground paprika, cumin & coriander
- ½ tsp ground ginger
- Low cal cooking oil spray
- Salt & pepper to taste

Method

1 Turn the slow cooker on so that it starts heating up.

2 Place a non-stick frying pan on a low heat and gently sauté the onions & in a little low cal spray for a few minutes until softened.

3 Tip the onions out of the pan onto a plate.

4 Add some more oil to the pan, increase the heat and quickly brown the lamb for a minute or two to seal the meat.

5 Add everything to the slow cooker. Combine well, cover with the lid and leave to cook on low for 5-6 hours or until the lamb is tender (add a little chicken stock if you need to during cooking)

6 When the stew is cooked through, check the seasoning and serve.

CHEFS NOTE
Add the sweet potatoes half way through cooking if you'd rather they stayed whole.

MOROCCAN MEATBALLS

300 calories per serving

Ingredients

- 1 onion, sliced
- 3 garlic cloves, crushed
- 500g/1lb 2oz lean minced beef
- 2 tbsp breadcrumbs
- 1 egg
- 1 cinnamon stick
- 3 tbsp tomato puree

- 1 tin chopped tomatoes (400g/14oz)
- 1 tsp paprika
- 6 dried apricots, finely chopped
- ½ tsp each salt & brown sugar
- Low cal cooking oil spray
- Salt & pepper to taste

Method

1 Turn the slow cooker on so that it starts heating up.

2 Place a non-stick frying pan on a low heat and gently sauté the onions & garlic in a little low cal spray for a few minutes until softened.

3 Meanwhile make breadcrumbs by taking the end crust from a loaf of bread and grate. Combine together the beef, breadcrumbs & egg (use a mixer if you've got one, use your hands if not).

4 Once everything is well combined shape into about 16-18 small firm meatballs.

5 Add everything to the slow cooker. Combine well, cover with the lid and leave to cook on low for 5-6 hours or high for 3-4 hours (give the meatballs a stir once or twice during cooking to keep them covered in sauce).

6 Check the seasoning of the sauce, remove the cinnamon stick and serve.

CHEFS NOTE
Serve with couscous and/or flat bread.

ROGAN LAMB

355
calories per serving

Ingredients

- 4 onions, sliced
- 2 garlic cloves, crushed
- 600g/1lb 5oz lean lamb leg or shoulder, cubed
- 60ml/¼ cup chicken stock
- 1 tin chopped tomatoes (400g/14oz)
- 2 red or green chillies, deseeded & finely chopped

- 3 tbsp tomato puree
- 1 tsp each turmeric, coriander, garam masala & cumin
- ½ tsp each ground ginger, salt & brown sugar
- Low cal cooking oil spray
- Salt & pepper to taste

Method

1 Turn the slow cooker on so that it starts heating up.

2 Place a non-stick frying pan on a low heat and gently sauté the onions & garlic in a little low cal spray for a few minutes until softened.

3 Tip the onions out of the pan onto a plate.

4 Add some more oil to the pan, increase the heat and quickly brown the lamb for a minute or two to seal the meat.

5 Add everything to the slow cooker. Combine well, cover with the lid and leave to cook on low for 5-6 hours or until the lamb is tender (add a little more stock if you need to during cooking).

6 When the stew is cooked through, check the seasoning and serve.

CHEFS NOTE
Use chilli powder if you don't have fresh chillies.

BEEF KOFTA

360
calories per serving

Ingredients

- 1 onion, sliced
- 2 garlic cloves, crushed
- 2 red or green peppers, deseeded & sliced
- 500g/1lb 2oz lean minced beef
- 2 tbsp breadcrumbs
- 1 tsp ground coriander

- 1 egg
- 3 tbsp tomato puree
- 500ml/2 cups tomato passata
- 2 tbsp curry powder
- Pinch of salt & brown sugar
- Low cal cooking oil spray
- Salt & pepper to taste

Method

1 Turn the slow cooker on so that it starts heating up.

2 Place a non-stick frying pan on a low heat and gently sauté the onions, garlic & peppers in a little low cal spray for a few minutes until softened.

3 Meanwhile make breadcrumbs by taking the end crust from a loaf of bread and grate. Combine together the beef, breadcrumbs, coriander & egg (use a mixer if you've got one, use your hands if not).

4 Once everything is well combined shape into about 16-18 small firm meatballs.

5 Add everything to the slow cooker. Combine well, cover with the lid and leave to cook on low for 5-6 hours or high for 3-4 hours (give the meatballs a stir once or twice during cooking to keep them covered in sauce).

6 Check the seasoning of the sauce and serve piled over rice.

CHEFS NOTE
Increase the 'heat' with fresh chillies if you like.

Skinny
SLOW COOKER
Student
VEGGIE DISHES

TURMERIC DAL

320 calories per serving

Ingredients

- 300g/11oz yellow split peas
- 1 onion, sliced
- 2 garlic cloves, crushed
- 2 red or orange peppers, deseeded & sliced
- 1 red chilli, deseeded & finely chopped
- 1 tsp ground cumin

- 2 tsp turmeric
- ½ tsp ground ginger
- 750ml/3 cups hot vegetable stock
- 1 lemon
- Low cal cooking oil spray
- Salt & pepper to taste

Method

1 Turn the slow cooker on so that it starts heating up.

2 Place a non-stick frying pan on a low heat and gently sauté the onions, garlic & peppers in a little low cal spray for a few minutes until softened.

3 Put everything in the slow cooker. Combine well, cover with the lid and leave to cook on low for 5-6 hours or high for 3-4 hours. Check the split peas are tender and the stock has been absorbed (add a little more during cooking if needed).

4 Cut the lemon into wedges and serve the dal with a squeeze of juice on top.

CHEFS NOTE

Fresh chopped coriander makes a good addition to this simple dal along with a dollop of cooling fat free Greek yogurt.

3 BEAN TAGINE

245 calories per serving

Ingredients

- 1 onion, chopped
- 2 garlic cloves, crushed
- 2 red or orange peppers, deseeded & sliced
- 1 red chilli, deseeded & finely chopped
- ½ tin chopped tomatoes (200g/7oz)
- 2 tbsp tomato puree

- 120ml/½ cup hot vegetable stock
- 1 tsp each ground coriander & paprika
- 2 tins mixed beans (800g/1¾lb), drained
- 2 tsp turmeric
- 1 courgette (200g/7oz)
- Low cal cooking oil spray
- Salt & pepper to taste

Method

1 Turn the slow cooker on so that it starts heating up.

2 Place a non-stick frying pan on a low heat and gently sauté the onions, garlic & peppers in a little low cal spray for a few minutes until softened.

3 Put everything, except the courgette, in the slow cooker. Combine well, cover with the lid and leave to cook on high for 2-4 hours, or until everything is cooked through and piping hot (cook for a little longer with the lid off if you need to thicken the sauce).

4 When the beans are ready take the courgette and 'julienne' with a potato peeler. This is basically turning the courgette into very fine ribbons, discard the fleshy core.

5 Load the beans into shallow bowls and sit the fine courgette ribbons on top.

CHEFS NOTE

Make the raw courgette ribbons as thin as you can and they will add a lovely fresh crunch to this dish.

MUSHROOM RISOTTO

330 calories per serving

Ingredients

- 1 onion, chopped
- 1 garlic clove, crushed
- 1 tbsp olive oil
- 300g/11oz risotto rice
- 1 tsp dried rosemary

- 1 punnet mushrooms (300g/11oz), sliced
- 1lt/4 cups vegetable stock
- Low cal cooking oil spray
- Salt & pepper to taste

Method

1 Turn the slow cooker on so that it starts heating up.

2 Place a large non-stick frying pan on a low heat and gently sauté the onions & garlic in the olive oil for a few minutes until softened.

3 Add the rice & rosemary and stir well to coat each rice grain in the oil.

4 Put everything in the slow cooker. Combine well, cover with the lid and leave to cook on high for 2-4 hours or until the risotto is tender and the stock has been absorbed (add a little more during cooking if needed).

5 Season and serve.

CHEFS NOTE
If you don't have rosemary use dried thyme or mixed herbs instead.

SQUASH & CHICKPEA ONE-POT

450 calories per serving

Ingredients

- 1 onion, chopped
- 2 garlic cloves, crushed
- 1 butternut squash (700g/1lb 9oz), peeled, deseeded & cubed
- ½ tin chopped tomatoes (200g/7oz)
- 2 tbsp tomato puree
- 120ml/½ cup hot vegetable stock

- 1 tsp each ground ginger, cumin & paprika
- 2 tins chickpeas, drained (800g/1lb 5oz)
- Low cal cooking oil spray
- Salt & pepper to taste

Method

1 Turn the slow cooker on so that it starts heating up.

2 Place a non-stick frying pan on a low heat and gently sauté the onions, garlic & squash in a little low cal spray for a few minutes until softened.

3 Put everything in the slow cooker. Combine well, cover with the lid and leave to cook on high for 2-4 hours, or until everything is cooked through and the squash is tender (cook for a little longer with the lid off if you need to thicken the sauce).

4 Check the seasoning and serve.

CHEFS NOTE
You could add a teaspoon of honey to give some unexpected sweetness to this savoury dish.

INDIAN CHICKPEA SAAG

199 calories per serving

Ingredients

- 1 onion, chopped
- 2 garlic cloves, crushed
- 1 tbsp curry powder
- 1 tin chopped tomatoes (400g/14oz)
- 2 tbsp tomato puree
- 120ml/½ cup hot vegetable stock
- 1½ tins chickpeas (600g/1lb 5oz), drained
- 4 handfuls spinach leaves (200g/7oz)
- Low cal cooking oil spray
- Salt & pepper to taste

Method

1 Turn the slow cooker on so that it starts heating up.

2 Prepare all the ingredients and put everything in the slow cooker.

3 Combine well, cover with the lid and leave to cook on high for 2-4 hours, or until everything is cooked through and piping hot.

4 Check the seasoning and serve.

CHEFS NOTE
This is especially good eaten with flatbread or naan bread.

GARLIC LENTIL STEW

385
calories per serving

Ingredients

- 300g/11oz red lentils
- 2 onion, sliced
- 4 garlic cloves, crushed
- 1 butternut squash (700g/1lb 9oz) peeled, deseeded & cubed
- 1 tbsp curry powder
- 750ml/3 cups hot vegetable stock
- 2 tbsp fat free Greek yogurt
- Low cal cooking oil spray
- Salt & pepper to taste

Method

1 Turn the slow cooker on so that it starts heating up.

2 Place a non-stick frying pan on a low heat and gently sauté the onions & garlic in a little low cal spray for a few minutes until softened.

3 Put everything, except the yogurt, in the slow cooker. Combine well, cover with the lid and leave to cook on low for 5-6 hours or high for 3-4 hours. Make sure the lentils & squash are tender and the stock has been absorbed (add a little more during cooking if needed).

4 When the stew is ready quickly stir through the yogurt and serve.

CHEFS NOTE

Cheap and easy to make, this stew is great for sharing with friends.

PEA & LEMON RISOTTO

330
calories per serving

Ingredients

- 2 onions, chopped
- 2 garlic cloves, crushed
- 1 tbsp olive oil
- 300g/11oz risotto rice
- 1lt/4 cups vegetable stock

- 4 handfuls frozen peas (200g/7oz)
- 1 lemon
- Low cal cooking oil spray
- Salt & pepper to taste

Method

1 Turn the slow cooker on so that it starts heating up.

2 Place a large non-stick frying pan on a low heat and gently sauté the onions & garlic in the olive oil for a few minutes until softened.

3 Add the rice and stir well to coat each rice grain in the oil.

4 Put everything, except the lemon, in the slow cooker. Combine well, cover with the lid and leave to cook on high for 2-4 hours. Check the risotto is tender and the stock has been absorbed (add a little more during cooking if needed).

5 Cut the lemon into wedges are serve the risotto with a squeeze of juice on top.

CHEFS NOTE
Grated vegetarian hard cheese makes a good addition to this perky risotto.

COURGETTE & CHERRY TOMATO TORTILLA

270 calories per serving

Ingredients

- 1 punnet cherry tomatoes (300g/11oz), halved
- 1 red onion, sliced
- 1 red or orange peppers, deseeded & sliced
- 2 courgettes (400g/14oz), diced
- 2 tbsp water
- 2 handfuls (100g/3½oz) peas
- 8 medium free range eggs
- Low cal cooking oil spray
- Salt & pepper to taste

Method

1 Turn the slow cooker on so that it starts heating up.

2 Put the tomatoes, onion, peppers, courgettes & water in the slow cooker. Combine well, cover with the lid and leave to cook on high for 1-2 hours or until tender.

3 Break the eggs into a bowl. Gently beat and season well. Scoop the veg out of the slow cooker and tip into the egg bowl.

4 Combine well and add everything back to the slow cooker (spray with some oil to prevent sticking).

5 Cover and leave to cook for another hour, or until the eggs are set and the vegetables cooked through.

6 Gently lift out of the cooker and serve sliced into thick wedges.

CHEFS NOTE

Serve with a simple green salad and low fat mayonnaise.

SWEET POTATO STEW

390 calories per serving

Ingredients

- 1 onion, sliced
- 2 garlic cloves, crushed
- 2 red or orange peppers, deseeded & sliced
- 1 red chilli, deseeded & finely chopped
- 60ml/¼ cup vegetable stock
- 2 tsp paprika
- 1 tin chopped tomatoes (400g/14oz)

- 4 sweet potatoes (1kg/2¼lb)
- 2 tbsp fat free Greek yogurt
- Low cal cooking oil spray
- Salt & pepper to taste

Method

1 Turn the slow cooker on so that it starts heating up.

2 Place a non-stick frying pan on a low heat and gently sauté the onions, garlic & peppers in a little low cal spray for a few minutes until softened.

3 Put everything, except the yogurt, in the slow cooker. Combine well, cover with the lid and leave to cook on high for 3-4 hours or until the sweet potatoes are tender.

4 Serve in shallow bowls and dollop the yogurt on top.

CHEFS NOTE
Sprinkle a little extra paprika over the yogurt if you like.

VEGGIE RATATOUILLE

195
calories per serving

Ingredients

- 1 onion, sliced
- 1 garlic clove, crushed
- 2 red or orange peppers, deseeded & sliced
- 2 aubergines
- 3 handfuls sweetcorn (150g/5oz)
- 60ml/¼ cup vegetable stock
- 2 tins chopped tomatoes (800g/1¾lb)

- 2 tbsp tomato puree
- ½ tsp salt & brown sugar
- 1 tsp dried oregano or basil
- Low cal cooking oil spray
- Salt & pepper to taste

Method

1 Turn the slow cooker on so that it starts heating up.

2 Place a non-stick frying pan on a low heat and gently sauté the onions, garlic & peppers in a little low cal spray for a few minutes until softened.

3 Top & tail the aubergines and cube the flesh - don't peel them.

4 Put everything in the slow cooker. Combine well, cover with the lid and leave to cook on high for 3-4 hours or low for 5-7 hours.

5 Check the seasoning and serve.

CHEFS NOTE
Feel free to throw in whatever veggies you have to hand.

77

BIRYANI

335
calories per
serving

Ingredients

- 1 onion, sliced
- 2 garlic cloves, crushed
- 1 red or orange peppers, deseeded & sliced
- 4 handfuls frozen peas (200g/7oz)
- 1 punnet mushrooms (300g/11oz), sliced
- 300g/11oz rice
- 500ml/2 cups hot vegetable stock
- 1 tbsp curry powder
- 1 red chilli, deseeded & very finely sliced
- Low cal cooking oil spray
- Salt & pepper to taste

Method

1 Turn the slow cooker on so that it starts heating up.

2 Place a non-stick frying pan on a low heat and gently sauté the onions, garlic & peppers in a little low cal spray for a few minutes until softened.

3 Put everything, except the sliced chilli, in the slow cooker. Combine well, cover with the lid and leave to cook on high for 2-4 hours. Check the rice is tender and the stock has been absorbed (add a little more during cooking if needed).

4 Sprinkle the finely sliced chillies over the top and serve.

CHEFS NOTE
Use red onion or thin slices of pepper if you don't want to garnish with chillies.

BARLEY STEW

195 calories per serving

Ingredients

- 1 onion, sliced
- 2 garlic cloves, crushed
- 1 red or orange peppers, deseeded & sliced
- 1 tsp each ground coriander, cumin & paprika
- 3 medium carrots (400g/14oz), peeled & sliced into batons
- 2 handfuls green beans (200g/7oz), chopped
- 250ml/1 cup hot vegetable stock
- 1 tin chopped tomatoes (400g/14oz)
- 125g/4oz pearl barley
- 1 tbsp tomato puree
- Low cal cooking oil spray
- Salt & pepper to taste

Method

1 Turn the slow cooker on so that it starts heating up.

2 Place a non-stick frying pan on a low heat and gently sauté the onions, garlic & peppers in a little low cal spray for a few minutes until softened.

3 Put everything in the slow cooker. Combine well, cover with the lid and leave to cook on high for 2-4 hours. Check the barley is tender and the stock has been absorbed (add a little more during cooking if needed). Season and serve.

CHEFS NOTE
Pearl barley is a traditional base for soups and stews.

BOSTON BEANS

250
calories per
serving

Ingredients

- 1 red onion, sliced
- 2 tsp brown sugar
- 2 garlic cloves, crushed
- ½ tin (200g/7oz) chopped tomatoes
- 120ml/½ cup hot vegetable stock
- 2 tins flageolet beans (800g/1¾lb), rinsed
- 1 tbsp Dijon mustard
- 2 tbsp ketchup
- Low cal cooking oil spray
- Salt & pepper to taste

Method

1 Turn the slow cooker on so that it starts heating up.

2 Place a non-stick frying pan on a low heat and gently sauté the red onions, garlic & sugar in a little low cal spray for a minute or two to caramelise the onions (don't let the sugar burn).

3 Put everything in the slow cooker. Combine well, cover with the lid and leave to cook on high for 2-3 hours or low for 4-5 hours or until everything is cooked through and piping hot.

4 Check the seasoning and serve.

CHEFS NOTE
Add a little chilli too if you like.

SERVES 4

MEXICAN CHILLI

275
calories per
serving

Ingredients

- 1 onion
- 3 medium carrots (400g/14oz)
- 4 tbsp ketchup
- 1 tbsp balsamic vinegar
- 1 tsp each ground cumin, chilli powder & dried oregano
- 120ml/½ cup hot vegetable stock
- 2 tins kidney beans (800g/1¾lb), rinsed
- Low cal cooking oil spray
- Salt & pepper to taste

Method

1 Turn the slow cooker on so that it starts heating up.

2 If you have a food processor use it to chop the onion and carrots very finely (if not you'll need to do the best you can by hand).

3 Place a non-stick frying pan on a low heat and gently sauté the chopped onions & carrots in a little low cal spray for a few minutes to soften (add a splash of water to the pan if you need to).

4 Put everything in the slow cooker. Combine well, cover with the lid and leave to cook on high for 2-3 hours or low for 4-5 hours or until everything is tender and cooked through.

5 Check the seasoning and serve.

CHEFS NOTE
Chopping the carrots and onions finely makes a base for the chilli to give it additional substance.

81

REAL DEAL MACARONI

490 calories per serving

Ingredients

- 1 tbsp Dijon mustard
- 120ml/½ cup evaporated milk
- 270ml/1½ cups semi skimmed milk
- 2 free range eggs
- 300g/11oz macaroni pasta
- 200g/7oz grated vegetarian reduced fat mature cheddar cheese
- 2 large tomatoes, sliced
- Low cal cooking oil spray
- Salt & pepper to taste

Method

1 Turn the slow cooker on so that it starts heating up.

2 Beat together the eggs, mustard, evaporated and semi skimmed milk.

3 Put everything in the slow cooker, except the tomatoes, in the slow cooker and combine well.

4 Arrange the tomato slices on top and leave to cook on high for 1½-2 hours or low for 2-3 hours, or until the pasta is tender and cooked through.

CHEFS NOTE
Keep an eye on the macaroni during cooking and add more milk if you need to.

Skinny
SLOW COOKER
Student
SEAFOOD DISHES

THAI FISH

295
calories per
serving

Ingredients

- 600g/1lb 5oz skinless, boneless white fish fillets
- 2 onions, sliced
- 2 garlic cloves, crushed
- 2 tbsp Thai green curry paste
- 1 tbsp tomato puree
- 380ml/1½ cups low fat coconut milk
- 4 handfuls frozen peas (200g/7oz)
- Low cal cooking oil spray
- Salt & pepper to taste

Method

1 Turn the slow cooker on so that it starts heating up.

2 Place a non-stick frying pan on a low heat and gently sauté the onions & garlic in a little low cal spray for a few minutes until softened.

3 Put everything in the slow cooker. Combine well, cover with the lid and leave to cook on high for 1-2 hours or until the fish is cooked through.

4 Season and serve with boiled rice or noodles.

CHEFS NOTE
Use whichever is the cheapest meaty white fish you can get your hands on.

HOT LIME FISH

225
calories per
serving

Ingredients

- 600g/1lb 5oz skinless, boneless white fish fillets, cubed
- 1 onion, sliced
- 2 red chillies, deseeded & finely sliced
- 4 garlic cloves, crushed
- 1 tsp each paprika, cumin & turmeric
- ½ tin (200g/7oz) chopped tomatoes
- 1 handful (200g/7oz) new potatoes,
- thickly sliced
- 1 tbsp tomato puree
- 120ml/½ cup chicken stock
- 2 tbsp lime juice
- 1 lime
- Low cal cooking oil spray
- Salt & pepper to taste

Method

1 Turn the slow cooker on so that it starts heating up.

2 Place a non-stick frying pan on a low heat and gently sauté the onions, chillies & garlic a little low cal spray for a few minutes until softened.

3 Put everything, except the whole lime, in the slow cooker. Combine well, cover with the lid and leave to cook on high for 1-2 hours or until the fish is cooked through and the potatoes are tender.

4 Cut the lime into wedges, load up the stew in shallow bowls, season and serve with the lime on the side.

CHEFS NOTE
Try serving with some raw sliced red onion and/or peppers on top of the stew.

TUNA NOODLES

400
calories per serving

Ingredients

- 300g/11oz fine egg noodles
- 2 onions, sliced
- 1 garlic clove, crushed
- 2 tins tuna (400g/7oz), drained
- 1 tin condensed mushroom soup

- (300g/11oz)
- 4 handfuls frozen peas (200g/7oz)
- Low cal cooking oil spray
- Salt & pepper to taste

Method

1 Turn the slow cooker on so that it starts heating up.

2 Boil the kettle, place the egg noodles in a bowl, cover with boiling water and leave to sit for a few minutes.

3 Meanwhile place a non-stick frying pan on a low heat and gently sauté the onions & garlic in a little low cal spray for a few minutes until softened.

4 Drain the noodles (reserve the water).

5 Put everything in the slow cooker. Half fill the empty soup tin with the drained noodle water and add to the slow cooker too. Combine well, cover with the lid and leave to cook on high for 1-2 hours or until the fish is cooked through.

6 Season and serve.

CHEFS NOTE
Quick and easy to make, add some grated Parmesan cheese if you wish.

FISH & RICE STEW

355 calories per serving

Ingredients

- 600g/1lb 5oz skinless, boneless white fish fillets, cubed
- 1 onion, sliced
- 1 tbsp tomato puree
- 1 tsp dried oregano and paprika
- 1 tin chopped tomatoes (400g/14oz)
- 500ml/2 cups hot chicken stock
- 200g/7oz long grain rice
- Low cal cooking oil spray
- Salt & pepper to taste

Method

1 Turn the slow cooker on so that it starts heating up.

2 Place a non-stick frying pan on a low heat and gently sauté the onions & garlic in a little low cal spray for a few minutes until softened.

3 Put everything in the slow cooker. Combine well, cover with the lid and leave to cook on high for 1-2 hours or until the fish is cooked through, the rice is tender and the stock has been absorbed (add more stock during cooking if you need to).

4 Season and serve with lots of black pepper.

CHEFS NOTE

You could also use salmon or prawns for this recipe if your budget can stretch to it.

FIVE SPICE FISH

195
calories per
serving

Ingredients

- 600g/1lb 5oz skinless, boneless white fish fillets, cubed
- 1 tbsp plain flour
- 2 tsp Chinese five spice powder
- 1 onion, sliced
- 1 garlic clove, crushed
- 1 tsp freshly grated ginger
- 2 red peppers, deseeded & sliced
- 250ml/1 cup chicken stock
- Low cal cooking oil spray
- Salt & pepper to taste

Method

1 Turn the slow cooker on so that it starts heating up.

2 Place the fish, flour and five spice powder in a small plastic bag and shake until the fish is covered.

3 Place a non-stick frying pan on a low heat and gently sauté the onions, garlic, ginger & peppers in a little low cal spray for a few minutes until softened.

4 Tip the onions and peppers onto a plate, add a little more oil to the frying pan and quickly seal the floured fish cubes for a minute or two.

5 Carefully put everything in the slow cooker. Gently combine, cover with the lid and leave to cook on high for 1-2 hours or until the fish is cooked through.

6 Season and serve.

CHEFS NOTE

Good with steamed rice or beansprouts this simple stew benefits from the unique taste of Chinese five spice powder.

MOROCCAN FISH STEW

390 calories per serving

Ingredients

- 600g/1lb 5oz skinless, boneless white fish fillets, cubed
- 1 tbsp plain flour
- 1 onion, sliced
- 1 garlic clove, crushed
- 1 tsp each ground coriander, cumin & paprika
- 1 cinnamon stock

- 2 tbsp pitted olives, sliced
- 2 tbsp tomato puree
- 3 large potatoes (750g/1lb 11oz), peeled & cubed into 2cm chunks
- 250ml/1 cup hot chicken stock
- Low cal cooking oil spray
- Salt & pepper to taste

Method

1 Turn the slow cooker on so that it starts heating up.

2 Place the fish & flour in a small plastic bag and shake until the fish is covered.

3 Place a non-stick frying pan on a low heat and gently sauté the onions & garlic in a little low cal spray for a few minutes until softened.

4 Tip the onions onto a plate, add a little more oil to the frying pan and quickly seal the floured fish cubes for a minute or two.

5 Carefully put everything in the slow cooker. Gently combine, cover with the lid and leave to cook on high for 1-2 hours or until the fish is cooked through and the potatoes are tender (add more stock during cooking if needed).

6 Remove the cinnamon stick, season the stew and serve.

CHEFS NOTE
Great served with freshly chopped flat leaf parsley or coriander.

FENNEL & RED WINE STEW

215 calories per serving

Ingredients

- 600g/1lb 5oz skinless, boneless white fish fillets, cubed
- 1 onion, sliced
- 2 garlic cloves, crushed
- ½ tsp fennel seeds
- 120ml/½ cup red wine
- Pinch dried crushed chillies
- 1 tin chopped tomatoes (400g/14oz)
- 1 tbsp tomato puree
- 120ml/½ cup fish or chicken stock
- Low cal cooking oil spray
- Salt & pepper to taste

Method

1 Turn the slow cooker on so that it starts heating up.

2 Place a non-stick frying pan on a low heat and gently sauté the onions, garlic & fennel seeds in a little low cal spray for a few minutes until softened. Add the red wine, increase the heat and leave on a hard simmer until the wine has reduced by half.

3 Put everything in the slow cooker. Combine well, cover with the lid and leave to cook on high for 1-2 hours or until the fish is cooked through.

4 Season and serve.

CHEFS NOTE

Try serving this stew loaded over thick hand cut slices of toasted white bread.

CHERRY TOMATO & PRAWN BURRIDA

235 calories per serving

Ingredients

- 1 onion, sliced
- 3 carrots (400g/14oz), peeled & diced
- 6 garlic cloves, crushed
- 1 punnet ripe cherry tomatoes (300g/11oz), halved
- 600g/1lb 5oz raw, shelled king prawns

- 250ml/1 cup fish stock
- 2 tbsp tomato puree
- 1 tsp dried thyme
- 120ml/½ cup fish stock
- Low cal cooking oil spray
- Salt & pepper to taste

Method

1 Turn the slow cooker on so that it starts heating up.

2 Place a large non-stick frying pan on a low heat and gently sauté the onions, carrots & garlic in a little low cal spray for a few minutes until softened. Add the cherry tomatoes and gently cook for 5 minutes longer.

3 Put everything in the slow cooker. Combine well, cover with the lid and leave to cook on high for 1-2 hours or until the fish is cooked through.

4 Season and serve in shallow bowls.

CHEFS NOTE
Mop of the lovely juices of this soup with thick slices of a French bread stick.

CREAMY PRAWN STEW

180
calories per
serving

Ingredients

- 2 celery stalks, sliced
- 1 onion, sliced
- 2 garlic cloves, crushed
- 120ml/½ cup white wine
- 1 tbsp cornflour, dissolved in a little warm water to make a paste

- 600g/1lb 5oz raw, shelled king prawns
- 120ml/½ cup fish or chicken stock
- 3 tbsp fat free crème fraiche
- Low cal cooking oil spray
- Salt & pepper to taste

Method

1 Turn the slow cooker on so that it starts heating up.

2 Place a non-stick frying pan on a low heat and gently sauté the celery, onions & garlic in a little low cal spray for a few minutes until softened. Add the wine, increase the heat and leave to cook on a hard simmer until the wine has reduced by half.

3 Stir through the cornflower paste and put everything, except the crème fraiche, in the slow cooker. Combine well, cover with the lid and leave to cook on high for 1-2 hours or until the fish is cooked through.

4 Stir through the crème fraiche, season and serve.

CHEFS NOTE
Bulk this dish up by adding a couple of handfuls of whatever greens or vegetables you have to hand.

CHORIZO & SEAFOOD STEW

300 calories per serving

Ingredients

- 2 small chorizo sausages (100g/3½oz), finely chopped
- 1 onion, sliced
- 2 garlic cloves, crushed
- 1 red chilli, deseeded & finely chopped
- 300g/11oz skinless, boneless white fish fillets, cubed
- 300g/11oz raw, shelled king prawns
- 1 tsp paprika
- 1 tbsp ground almonds
- 2 tbsp tomato puree
- 250ml/1 cup fish or chicken stock
- Low cal cooking oil spray
- Salt & pepper to taste

Method

1 Turn the slow cooker on so that it starts heating up.

2 Place a non-stick frying pan on a low heat and gently sauté the onions, garlic & chilli in a little low cal spray for a few minutes until softened.

3 Carefully put everything in the slow cooker. Gently combine, cover with the lid and leave to cook on high for 1-2 hours or until the fish & prawns are cooked through.

4 Check the seasoning and serve.

CHEFS NOTE
Flaked almonds when serving make a great addition.

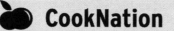 **CookNation**

Other COOKNATION TITLES

If you enjoyed 'The Skinny Slow Cooker Student Recipe Book' we'd really appreciate your feedback. Reviews help others decide if this is the right book for them so a moment of your time would be appreciated.

Thank you.

You may also be interested in other '**Skinny**' titles in the CookNation series. You can find all the following great titles by searching under '**CookNation**'.

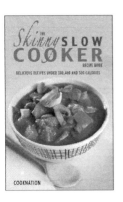

THE SKINNY SLOW COOKER RECIPE BOOK

Delicious Recipes Under 300, 400 And 500 Calories.

Paperback / eBook

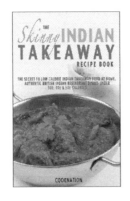

THE SKINNY INDIAN TAKEAWAY RECIPE BOOK

Authentic British Indian Restaurant Dishes Under 300, 400 And 500 Calories. The Secret To Low Calorie Indian Takeaway Food At Home.

Paperback / eBook

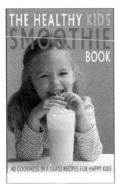

THE HEALTHY KIDS SMOOTHIE BOOK

40 Delicious Goodness In A Glass Recipes for Happy Kids.

eBook

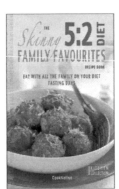

THE SKINNY 5:2 FAST DIET FAMILY FAVOURITES RECIPE BOOK

Eat With All The Family On Your Diet Fasting Days.

Paperback / eBook

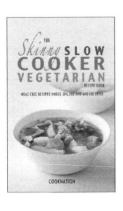

THE SKINNY SLOW COOKER VEGETARIAN RECIPE BOOK

40 Delicious Recipes Under 200, 300 And 400 Calories.

Paperback / eBook

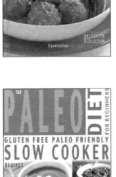

THE PALEO DIET FOR BEGINNERS SLOW COOKER RECIPE BOOK

Gluten Free, Everyday Essential Slow Cooker Paleo Recipes For Beginners.

eBook

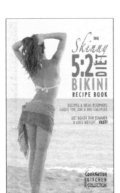

THE SKINNY 5:2 SLOW COOKER RECIPE BOOK

Skinny Slow Cooker Recipe And Menu Ideas Under 100, 200, 300 & 400 Calories For Your 5:2 Diet.

Paperback / eBook

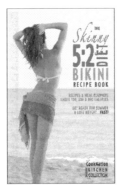

THE SKINNY 5:2 BIKINI DIET RECIPE BOOK

Recipes & Meal Planners Under 100, 200 & 300 Calories. Get Ready For Summer & Lose Weight...FAST!

Paperback / eBook

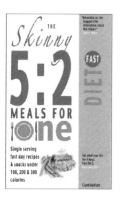

THE SKINNY 5:2 FAST DIET MEALS FOR ONE

Single Serving Fast Day Recipes & Snacks Under 100, 200 & 300 Calories.

Paperback / eBook

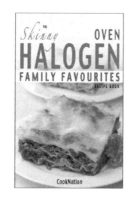

THE SKINNY HALOGEN OVEN FAMILY FAVOURITES RECIPE BOOK

Healthy, Low Calorie Family Meal-Time Halogen Oven Recipes Under 300, 400 and 500 Calories.

Paperback / eBook

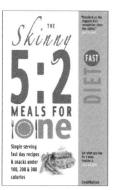

THE SKINNY 5:2 FAST DIET VEGETARIAN MEALS FOR ONE

Single Serving Fast Day Recipes & Snacks Under 100, 200 & 300 Calories.

Paperback / eBook

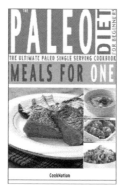

THE PALEO DIET FOR BEGINNERS MEALS FOR ONE

The Ultimate Paleo Single Serving Cookbook.

Paperback / eBook

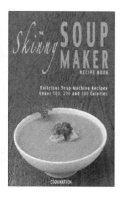

THE SKINNY SOUP MAKER RECIPE BOOK

Delicious Low Calorie, Healthy and Simple Soup Recipes Under 100, 200 and 300 Calories. Perfect For Any Diet and Weight Loss Plan.

Paperback / eBook

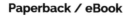

THE PALEO DIET FOR BEGINNERS HOLIDAYS

Thanksgiving, Christmas & New Year Paleo Friendly Recipes.
eBook

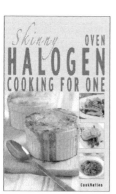

SKINNY HALOGEN OVEN COOKING FOR ONE

Single Serving, Healthy, Low Calorie Halogen Oven RecipesUnder 200, 300 and 400 Calories.

Paperback / eBook

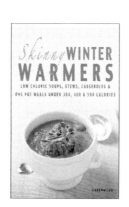

SKINNY WINTER WARMERS RECIPE BOOK

Soups, Stews, Casseroles & One Pot Meals Under 300, 400 & 500 Calories.

Paperback / eBook

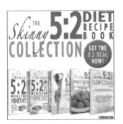

THE SKINNY 5:2 DIET RECIPE BOOK COLLECTION

All The 5:2 Fast Diet Recipes You'll Ever Need. All Under 100, 200, 300, 400 And 500 Calories.

eBook

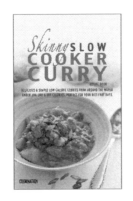

THE SKINNY SLOW COOKER CURRY RECIPE BOOK

Low Calorie Curries From Around The World.

Paperback / eBook

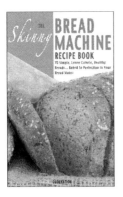

THE SKINNY BREAD MACHINE RECIPE BOOK

70 Simple, Lower Calorie, Healthy Breads...Baked To Perfection In Your Bread Maker.

Paperback / eBook

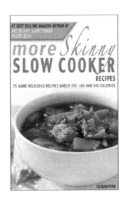

MORE SKINNY SLOW COOKER RECIPES

75 More Delicious Recipes Under 300, 400 & 500 Calories.

Paperback / eBook

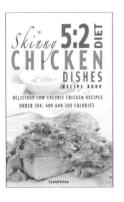

THE SKINNY 5:2 DIET CHICKEN DISHES RECIPE BOOK

Delicious Low Calorie Chicken Dishes Under 300, 400 & 500 Calories.

Paperback / eBook

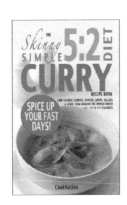

THE SKINNY 5:2 CURRY RECIPE BOOK

Spice Up Your Fast Days With Simple Low Calorie Curries, Snacks, Soups, Salads & Sides Under 200, 300 & 400 Calories.

Paperback / eBook

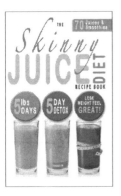

THE SKINNY JUICE DIET RECIPE BOOK

5lbs, 5 Days. The Ultimate Kick- Start Diet and Detox Plan to Lose Weight & Feel Great!

Paperback / eBook

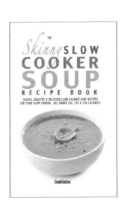

THE SKINNY SLOW COOKER SOUP RECIPE BOOK

Simple, Healthy & Delicious Low Calorie Soup Recipes For Your Slow Cooker. All Under 100, 200 & 300 Calories.

Paperback / eBook

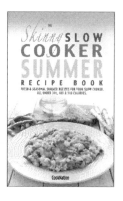

THE SKINNY SLOW COOKER SUMMER RECIPE BOOK

Fresh & Seasonal Summer Recipes For Your Slow Cooker. All Under 300, 400 And 500 Calories.

Paperback / eBook

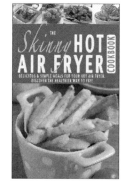

THE SKINNY HOT AIR FRYER COOKBOOK

Delicious & Simple Meals For Your Hot Air Fryer: Discover The Healthier Way To Fry.

Paperback / eBook

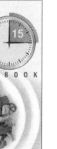

THE SKINNY ACTIFRY COOKBOOK

Guilt-free and Delicious ActiFry Recipe Ideas: Discover The Healthier Way to Fry!

Paperback / eBook

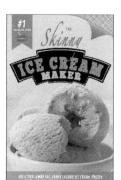

THE SKINNY ICE CREAM MAKER

Delicious Lower Fat, Lower Calorie Ice Cream, Frozen Yogurt & Sorbet Recipes For Your Ice Cream Maker.

Paperback / eBook

THE SKINNY 15 MINUTE MEALS RECIPE BOOK

Delicious, Nutritious & Super-Fast Meals in 15 Minutes Or Less. All Under 300, 400 & 500 Calories.

Paperback / eBook

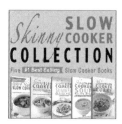

THE SKINNY SLOW COOKER COLLECTION

5 Fantastic Books of Delicious, Diet-friendly Skinny Slow Cooker Recipes: ALL Under 200, 300, 400 & 500 Calories!
eBook

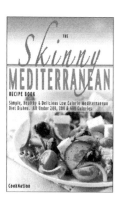

THE SKINNY MEDITERRANEAN RECIPE BOOK

Simple, Healthy & Delicious Low Calorie Mediterranean Diet Dishes. All Under 200, 300 & 400 Calories.

Paperback / eBook

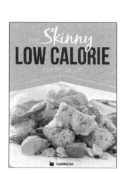

THE SKINNY LOW CALORIE RECIPE BOOK

Great Tasting, Simple & Healthy Meals Under 300, 400 & 500 Calories. Perfect For Any Calorie Controlled Diet.

Paperback / eBook

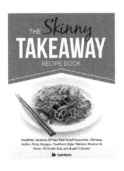

THE SKINNY TAKEAWAY RECIPE BOOK

Healthier Versions Of Your Fast Food Favourites: All Under 300, 400 & 500 Calories.

Paperback / eBook

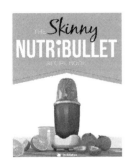

THE SKINNY NUTRIBULLET RECIPE BOOK

80+ Delicious & Nutritious Healthy Smoothie Recipes. Burn Fat, Lose Weight and Feel Great!

Paperback / eBook

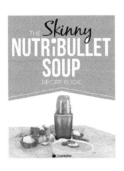

THE SKINNY NUTRIBULLET SOUP RECIPE BOOK

Delicious, Quick & Easy, Single Serving Soups & Pasta Sauces For Your Nutribullet. All Under 100, 200, 300 & 400 Calories!

Paperback / eBook

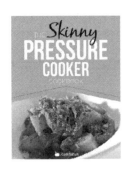

THE SKINNY PRESSURE COOKER COOKBOOK

USA ONLY

Low Calorie, Healthy & Delicious Meals, Sides & Desserts. All Under 300, 400 & 500 Calories.

Paperback / eBook

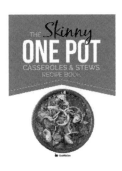

THE SKINNY ONE-POT RECIPE BOOK

Simple & Delicious, One-Pot Meals. All Under 300, 400 & 500 Calories

Paperback / eBook

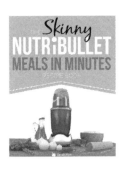

THE SKINNY NUTRIBULLET MEALS IN MINUTES RECIPE BOOK

Quick & Easy, Single Serving Suppers, Snacks, Sauces, Salad Dressings & More Using Your Nutribullet. All Under 300, 400 & 500 Calories

Paperback / eBook

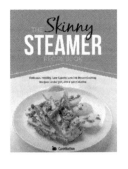

THE SKINNY STEAMER RECIPE BOOK

Healthy, Low Calorie, Low Fat Steam Cooking Recipes Under 300, 400 & 500 Calories.

Paperback / eBook

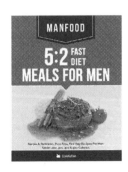

MANFOOD: 5:2 FAST DIET MEALS FOR MEN

Simple & Delicious, Fuss Free, Fast Day Recipes For Men Under 200, 300, 400 & 500 Calories.

Paperback / eBook

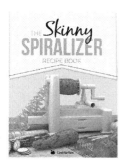

THE SKINNY SPIRALIZER RECIPE BOOK

Delicious Spiralizer Inspired Low Calorie Recipes For One. All Under 200, 300, 400 & 500 Calories

Paperback / eBook

CONVERSION CHART: DRY INGREDIENTS

Metric	Imperial
7g	¼ oz
15g	½ oz
20g	¾ oz
25g	1 oz
40g	1½oz
50g	2oz
60g	2½oz
75g	3oz
100g	3½oz
125g	4oz
140g	4½oz
150g	5oz
165g	5½oz
175g	6oz
200g	7oz
225g	8oz
250g	9oz
275g	10oz
300g	11oz
350g	12oz
375g	13oz
400g	14oz

Metric	Imperial
425g	15oz
450g	1lb
500g	1lb 2oz
550g	1¼lb
600g	1lb 5oz
650g	1lb 7oz
675g	1½lb
700g	1lb 9oz
750g	1lb 11oz
800g	1¾lb
900g	2lb
1kg	2¼lb
1.1kg	2½lb
1.25kg	2¾lb
1.35kg	3lb
1.5kg	3lb 6oz
1.8kg	4lb
2kg	4½lb
2.25kg	5lb
2.5kg	5½lb
2.75kg	6lb

CONVERSION CHART: LIQUID MEASURES

Metric	Imperial	US
25ml	1fl oz	
60ml	2fl oz	¼ cup
75ml	2½ fl oz	
100ml	3½fl oz	
120ml	4fl oz	½ cup
150ml	5fl oz	
175ml	6fl oz	
200ml	7fl oz	
250ml	8½ fl oz	1 cup
300ml	10½ fl oz	
360ml	12½ fl oz	
400ml	14fl oz	
450ml	15½ fl oz	
600ml	1 pint	
750ml	1¼ pint	3 cups
1 litre	1½ pints	4 cups

Printed in Great Britain
by Amazon